NATIONAL REPORT

WITHDRAWN

testing

times

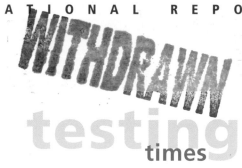

1 — Understanding Diabetes

Diabetes is a serious disease, accounting for significant and rising costs to the NHS.

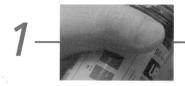

2² — Planning Services

Services are often poorly co-ordinated and may not meet the needs of different patient groups.

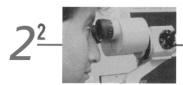

WITHDRAWN

3 — Delivering Effective Care

There is good evidence about what works in diabetes care, but many services fall short of best practice.

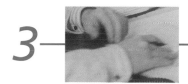

4 — Meeting the Challenges of the 21st Century

Hospital diabetes services need to re-focus their activity, to meet the dramatic increases in patient demands without compromising quality.

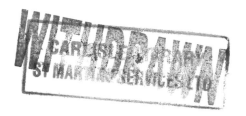

Contents

© Audit Commission 2000

First published in April 2000 by the Audit Commission for Local Authorities and
the National Health Service in England and Wales, 1 Vincent Square,
London SW1P 2PN

Printed in the UK for the Audit Commission by Belmont Press, Northampton

ISBN 1 86240 215 9

Photographs: Janis Austin/Photofusion (pp 16, 24), British Diabetes Association
(cover), Jacky Chapman/Format (p47), Lesley Howling/Collections (p7),
Crispin Hughes/Photofusion (p3), Ulrike Preuss/Format (p28), Hilary Shedel (p16),
Sam Tanner/Photofusion (p55), Mike Uttley (p96)

Preface

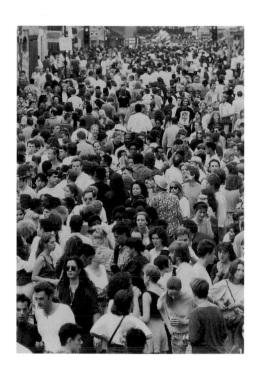

Diabetes is a serious disease which accounts for about 9 per cent of hospital costs, although total costs are much larger. It affects at least 3 per cent of the population, although many more are undiagnosed, and numbers are rising rapidly. There is no cure for diabetes and much of the burden of care falls on individuals who have to manage the disease themselves day to day. There is an increased risk of cardiovascular disease, kidney problems and serious complications affecting the eyes and feet – leading in some cases to blindness and amputation.

The good news is that there is sound evidence about what works. We know that good management can reduce the risk of serious complications and lengthen life. This means prompt diagnosis, regular checks to identify serious complications at an early stage, and treatment to control blood glucose and blood pressure levels. Support and education is crucial so that individuals can manage this complex disease effectively themselves.

But not all patients are receiving the best care. The Audit Commission carried out a study of diabetes services, focusing mainly on a small sample of hospitals in England and Wales, but also including surveys of health authorities, general practices and a large study of patients. The results showed variable levels of care, with many services struggling to cope with present demand. They will be under greater pressure as patient numbers rise. This report suggests how diabetes teams can re-focus their efforts to support staff in primary care and the community so that more routine care can be provided outside hospital settings.

As part of this study, auditors will work with hospitals in England and Wales over the coming year to review current services and improve patient care. Evidence from the audit and this report will help to inform the National Service Framework on diabetes, which will be published in spring 2001. This should raise the profile of diabetes care and set standards for services across the country.

Beverley Fitzsimons, Tara Lamont and Lesley Wilton from the Public Services Research Directorate of the Audit Commission carried out the study, under the direction of Anita Houghton and Ian Seccombe. Further input was provided by Linda Jarrett, with data analysis and support from Clare Hazard, Lucy McCulloch and Karen Wright. The audit approach was devised with help from Karen Smith and David Thomas. Members of a multi-disciplinary Advisory Group provided expert advice throughout the study and they are listed in Appendix II. As always, responsibility for the contents and conclusions rests solely with the Audit Commission.

Summary of key messages

I did not realise how serious diabetes was at first. Perhaps I might have taken it more seriously if I knew then what I know now.

Audit Commission survey of people with diabetes

Diabetes is a serious, lifelong disease that is known to affect at least 3 per cent of adults in the UK and accounts for about 9 per cent of total hospital costs. There is now good evidence to show that early diagnosis and good management can reduce the risk of premature death and complications, which include coronary heart disease, stroke, kidney failure, lower limb amputation, and blindness. These measures include better control of blood glucose and blood pressure and close monitoring of risk factors. Good support and education is essential so that people with diabetes can care for themselves. In the long term, empowering patients is the key to improving health and reducing demands on the service.

The Government is drawing up a National Service Framework for diabetes services, which is due to be published in 2001. This reflects the importance of the condition, in terms of costs both to the NHS and the individual.

Diabetes is common, costly, and increasing in prevalence.

- Diabetes affects about 3 per cent of the population – but up to half of people with diabetes are thought to be undiagnosed.

- The prevalence of diabetes increases with age and is three to four times more common in people of Asian and African-Caribbean origin.

- The number of people with diabetes in the UK is expected to increase from 1.4 million to 3 million by the year 2010 because of the ageing population and increasing levels of obesity.

- The total cost of diabetes care in this country is not known, but is likely to exceed £2 billion a year. Hospital costs are six times higher for a person with diabetes than for a person without diabetes.

- Hospital censuses for this study showed that from 6 to 16 per cent of beds are occupied by people with diabetes.

- Services are already stretched, with waiting times for first appointments up to 14 weeks and patient complaints of long clinic waits and insufficient time with staff.

There is clear evidence that good management reduces complications...

- Better blood glucose control reduces eye disease by one-quarter, and kidney disease by one-third.

- Effective eye screening and treatment can reduce blindness by half.

- Early intervention for foot problems can reduce amputations by two-thirds.
- Little cost-effectiveness research has been done, although there is clear evidence on what works in diabetes care.

I do feel I am a number and not a person with my own individual needs.

...but patients are not always receiving the best care.

- 20 per cent of patients said that they had insufficient access to advice when they needed it, and only two out of nine hospitals had formal arrangements for out of hours advice.
- Few hospitals had dedicated psychological support for people with diabetes.
- Less than half of the hospitals visited had comprehensive programmes of patient education, and two-thirds of patients surveyed said that they had received no education or support within the last 12 months.
- Almost half of the patients from ethnic minority groups reported understanding little or nothing about the effects of an illness like flu on their diabetes, and more than a quarter did not know what to expect if their blood glucose dropped too low.
- Two-thirds of hospitals visited could not produce information on how many patients had received a recent full review.

I have nobody to contact after hours and sometimes feel very alone with this.

More patients are now being managed in primary care, but standards vary.

- Primary care teams are now providing routine care for about 75 per cent of their patients with diabetes, with one-third of clinics run by practice nurses alone.
- Less than one-third of practices in the survey of general practices had routine access to a dietician or podiatrist (chiropodist).
- At one hospital foot clinic, half of the patients reviewed had been referred late from the community, and the general practice survey showed that over one-third of practices had no guidelines for diabetes referrals.

There is an urgent need for better strategic planning and monitoring to cope with rising demands.

- Less than one-quarter of health authorities had good quality population-based information on diabetes.
- Marked rises in patient numbers mean that current patterns of care need to be reviewed, yet less than half of health authorities surveyed had done this recently.

Conclusions

The prevalence of diabetes and the cost of providing services are likely to increase dramatically over the next ten years. Services are already under considerable strain, and little is taking place in the way of strategic planning. Options for coping with future demands need to be explored urgently. One way forward is for primary care to provide more routine care for people with diabetes, so that hospitals can concentrate on specialist care and professional support and training, while allowing patients to receive continuity of care closer to home. But staff in primary care need support to ensure consistently high quality services for patients. Primary care groups and local health groups provide a new opportunity for monitoring quality and raising standards in primary care.

This study is accompanied by a programme of audits of hospital diabetes services in England and Wales, which should help hospitals to assess their local services and prepare for the National Service Framework in 2001.

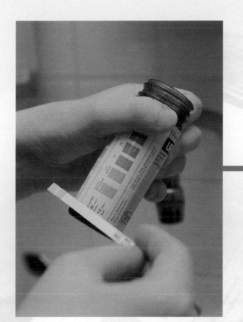

1

Understanding Diabetes

Diabetes is a serious disease, accounting for a significant and rising proportion of NHS spend. Patterns of care differ around the country and the role of the hospital diabetes team varies from place to place. There is good evidence on what treatments are effective and the last few decades have seen real improvements to patient care, with developments like specialist diabetes nurses. But not all patients may be benefiting from best practice.

Introduction

1. This is a critical time for diabetes services. Numbers of people with diabetes are increasing, new evidence is emerging on the effectiveness of more intensive treatment, patient expectations are rising and services are being stretched to their absolute limit. The question is, how can services cope with this rising demand?

2. While diabetes has traditionally been treated in hospitals, the last 20 years has seen a steady increase in the proportion of routine care provided in general practice and the community. But this has not happened everywhere, and patterns of care vary substantially across the country. Individuals are often seen in more than one setting, raising the potential for duplication and fragmentation, and poor communication across sectors has led to confusion and gaps in services.

3. Many of these problems are common to other chronic conditions, such as arthritis or asthma. But there is much better evidence in the field of diabetes about what works and a growing recognition of the serious nature of the disease (Ref. 1). The Government has identified diabetes as one of the first clinical areas for a National Service Framework. This will set national standards, define service models, put in place strategies to support implementation and delivery and establish performance measures against which progress will be monitored. The Framework is being developed now and should be published in 2001.

4. This study from the Audit Commission is therefore very timely. Based on research conducted at nine hospitals throughout the country, surveys of general practices, health authorities and patients, the report describes the current state of diabetes services. Case studies have been used to bring to life the problems facing both service users and staff, and to illustrate how good practice can be achieved. The report also considers the possible future direction of diabetes services, in the light of increasing demand.

5. This report is accompanied by a programme of local audits of hospital diabetes services in England and Wales during the year 2000. This work should provide useful evidence and baseline data for developing standards through the National Service Framework in 2001.

What is diabetes

6. Diabetes mellitus is a complex condition in which the body is unable to control the amount of sugar in the blood, either because there is an absence of the hormone insulin or because the insulin that is produced is not fully effective (Ref. 2). Uncontrolled diabetes can lead to metabolic disturbances that increase the risk of long-term complications affecting a number of the body's systems [BOX A].

BOX A

What is diabetes?

- A lifelong, chronic condition, characterised by the body's inability to control the amount of sugar in the blood.

- Diabetes affects about 3 per cent of the population – but many people remain undiagnosed, so the total number of people with diabetes may be much higher.

- Prevalence is much higher among elderly people and in some ethnic minority communities.

- It can lead to short term debilitating symptoms and long term major complications of heart, blood vessels, nerves, eyes and kidneys.

- Treating complications represents a major health service cost.

- The number of people with diabetes is predicted to rise dramatically – from 1.4 million to 3 million by the year 2010.

Source: Audit Commission

There is [good] evidence in the field of diabetes about what works and a growing recognition of the serious nature of the disease

7. In Type 1 (previously known as insulin dependent) diabetes, the pancreas produces insufficient insulin. It usually presents with symptoms of extreme tiredness and excessive thirst, and onset may be very rapid and result in acute emergency admission. Uncontrolled hyperglycaemia (raised blood glucose) can lead to ketoacidosis,[1] a serious condition which can cause multiple system failure and death.

8. Type 2 (previously known as non-insulin dependent) diabetes has complex causes, including reduced sensitivity to circulating insulin. It is more common and represents more than 80 per cent of cases of diabetes, with over a million people diagnosed in the UK. Onset is usually much slower than Type 1 diabetes, and patients may be asymptomatic for many years, only presenting when complications occur. People with Type 2 diabetes are sometimes mistakenly told that they have a 'mild' form of the condition, but research shows that Type 2 diabetes is as likely to cause serious complications as Type 1 (Ref. 1).

9. Complications associated with both types of diabetes include a higher risk of coronary heart disease, stroke, foot ulceration and amputation, kidney failure, neuropathy (nerve problems), diabetic retinopathy (eye disease) and blindness [EXHIBIT 1, overleaf].

---

[1] A glossary is given at the end of this report to explain terms like ketoacidosis, which may not be familiar to the general reader.

EXHIBIT 1

Complications of diabetes

Diabetes is associated with a range of serious complications.

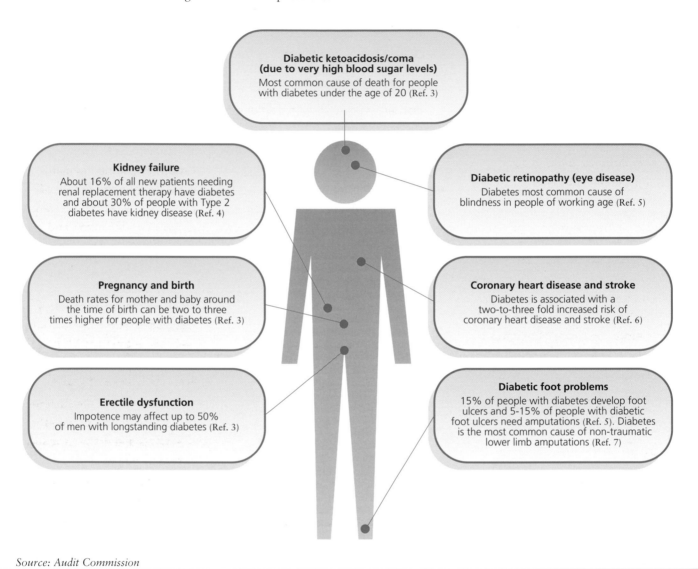

Diabetic ketoacidosis/coma (due to very high blood sugar levels)
Most common cause of death for people with diabetes under the age of 20 (Ref. 3)

Kidney failure
About 16% of all new patients needing renal replacement therapy have diabetes and about 30% of people with Type 2 diabetes have kidney disease (Ref. 4)

Diabetic retinopathy (eye disease)
Diabetes most common cause of blindness in people of working age (Ref. 5)

Pregnancy and birth
Death rates for mother and baby around the time of birth can be two to three times higher for people with diabetes (Ref. 3)

Coronary heart disease and stroke
Diabetes is associated with a two-to-three fold increased risk of coronary heart disease and stroke (Ref. 6)

Erectile dysfunction
Impotence may affect up to 50% of men with longstanding diabetes (Ref. 3)

Diabetic foot problems
15% of people with diabetes develop foot ulcers and 5-15% of people with diabetic foot ulcers need amputations (Ref. 5). Diabetes is the most common cause of non-traumatic lower limb amputations (Ref. 7)

Source: Audit Commission

10. Scientific developments and changes in service delivery, such as the emergence of specialist diabetes nurses, have changed the lives of people with diabetes over the last century **[BOX B]**. Before the identification of insulin in 1921, there was little treatment available for people with Type 1 diabetes. Treatment options now available mean that people with diabetes can live long and full lives. There is also greater understanding of the ways in which serious complications can be prevented and the importance of helping people to manage the condition effectively themselves.

BOX B

The changing face of diabetes care

Scientific advances and changes in the organisation of diabetes services have changed the lives of people with diabetes over recent decades. Critical landmarks include:

1920s

- Insulin identified and found to lower blood glucose in dogs. Subsequent tests on humans were successful and revolutionised the treatment for people with Type 1 diabetes.

1930s

- The Diabetic Association (later the British Diabetic Association) set up in the UK to campaign for universal access to insulin, before the National Health Service was established.
- Urine testing kits developed.
- First long-acting insulin produced.

1950s

- Diabetes and endocrinology established as medical specialties in their own right.

1970s

- Development of portable blood glucose meters enable people to monitor blood glucose at home.
- Development of laser treatment and eye screening services.

- Development (patchy) of diabetes centres in some hospitals, so that patients are not seen in general outpatient clinics.

1980s

- Development of diabetes specialist nurses as a profession.
- Development of diabetes multidisciplinary teams, including the expertise of podiatrists and dietitians as well as medical and nursing skills.
- St Vincent declaration (1989) raises the profile of diabetes internationally and sets targets for reducing complications.

1990s

- Many GPs set up mini-clinics as a result of changes in contracts and health promotion payments. This consolidated the shift of care, with many people with diabetes now being managed in general practice rather than hospital settings.
- Disposable syringes and 'pens' widely available for those injecting insulin.

- Landmark research trials (see Box E) demonstrate that good control reduces the risk of complications for people with diabetes.
- Local Diabetes Services Advisory Groups established in many areas, to raise the profile of diabetes services and convene a range of professionals and patients to shape services.

2000+

- The Government produces a National Service Framework for diabetes in the year 2001 to set standards for diabetes care across England and Wales.
- Development of primary care trusts changes the organisation of services and diabetes teams in some areas.
- Scientific advances may include non-invasive blood glucose monitoring, nasal or oral administration of insulin, gene therapy to identify people at risk of diabetes and its complications, artificial pancreas and other developments which may further transform the lives of people with diabetes.

Source: Audit Commission

Impact on society

Patient numbers

11. Diabetes is a serious chronic condition, which is known to affect about 3 per cent of the population. It is thought that up to half of all cases of diabetes may be undiagnosed, so the true prevalence may be much higher. In addition, prevalence is much higher in some population subgroups [**EXHIBIT 2**]. Ten per cent of people aged over 65 and more than one-quarter of people of Asian origin aged over 60 suffer from the condition (Ref. 3). The ageing of the population, especially in Asian and African-Caribbean communities, and marked increases in the rate of obesity mean that the absolute number of people with diabetes is set to grow substantially. Incidence is also rising among children under five years of age. Recent estimates suggest that, in the UK, the population with diabetes could rise from 1.4 million to 3 million by the year 2010 (Ref. 8). Recent changes in diagnostic criteria which lower the threshold for defining diabetes (Ref. 9) are also likely to result in increases in reported prevalence. Taken together, these trends mean substantial increases in demands for diabetes services.

EXHIBIT 2

Prevalence of diabetes in different ethnic groups

Diabetes is particularly common among Asian people*...

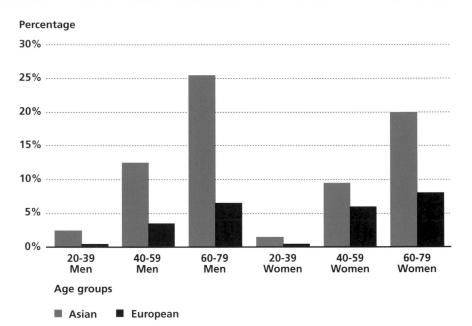

...and also for those of African-Caribbean origin (Ref. 10).

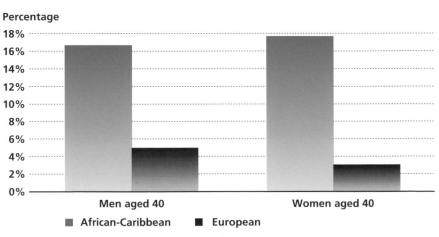

*Pooled data from four UK studies 1986-1993. Quoted in (Ref. 3).

Source: British Diabetic Association

Costs of diabetes care

12. Information on total costs of diabetes care is patchy,[1] especially on costs outside the hospital setting. But we know that resource use is greatest in the treatment of complications, which are the cause of high numbers of inpatient episodes and longer than average hospital stays for people with diabetes (Ref. 12). One 1988 study found that inpatient demands were five times those of people without diabetes (Ref. 13). A more recent study in 1996 showed that people with diabetes accounted for 5.4 per cent of all completed hospital episodes, 6.4 per cent of outpatient attendances and 9.4 per cent of inpatient bed days (Ref. 14). These figures show high levels of hospital use. But few studies have attempted to identify the overall costs of diabetes to society, including healthcare costs in primary and community settings and wider issues such as absence from work and loss of earnings.

13. In healthcare terms alone, costing diabetes services is extremely difficult. Diabetes is usually funded as part of the general medical budget in trusts, and because few members of staff are dedicated to diabetes, it is not possible to quantify with any accuracy the resources allocated to diabetes. Added to this, many of the conditions that people with diabetes suffer from are extremely common – for example, heart disease and stroke – so it is difficult to decide what proportion of these problems to ascribe to diabetes. Even if someone with diabetes is being treated in hospital for an entirely unrelated problem – for example, an elective hip operation – the presence of diabetes can complicate any medical or surgical procedure and therefore increase costs by lengthening the hospital stay.

14. For these reasons, one of the few studies (Currie et al.) attempting to cost diabetes services, decided to assess the total cost to the hospital for each person with diabetes in a district in South Wales, regardless of the reason for admission or attendance at hospital. They then assessed the average annual hospital expenditure per person without diabetes, thus calculating the excess cost due to the presence of diabetes. They arrived at a figure of around £2,100 per person with diabetes, and £300 per person without diabetes, giving an excess cost of approximately £1,800 per person with diabetes. Overall, they estimated that about 9 per cent of hospital costs are accounted for by people with diabetes (Ref. 15).

---

1   The only published estimate of total diabetes spend in the UK is of £1 billion in 1989 (Ref. 11) based on an estimate of 4-5 per cent of total healthcare expenditure, but this is likely to be somewhat outdated now, given recent evidence on service use by people with diabetes and what we know of current prevalence.

...diabetes is an area of significant and growing spend for the NHS...

15. Based on these south Wales figures of costs per patient, and given a current known prevalence of around 3 per cent, a district of 500,000 population would therefore be expected to spend around £30 million a year on hospital costs for people with diabetes. At a national level, an estimate of 9 per cent of UK hospital costs would lead to a figure of around £1.9 billion based on recent hospital returns.[1] However, as cost analyses for diabetes are so rare, it is impossible to know with any certainty how applicable the South Wales figures are to other districts. Moreover, these figures exclude non-hospital costs, although the bulk of routine diabetes care takes place in primary care settings. These estimates should therefore be viewed with caution and true costs are likely to be much higher overall.

16. But there is also the question of increasing demand as patient numbers rise, which will lead to greater levels of NHS spend. In addition, best available evidence indicates that intensive treatment is most effective in minimising the effects of complications (Ref. 16). This has resource implications, both in terms of increased treatment (for instance, greater use of anti-hypertensive drugs to control blood pressure) and staff costs (for instance, more specialist nursing input to support people switching to insulin). Even though authoritative evidence is not available on the total costs of diabetes care, it is clear that diabetes is an area of significant and growing spend for the NHS, which should be given high priority by clinicians, health service managers and policymakers.

Impact on individuals

17. Once people have been diagnosed with a chronic condition, they usually have to live with it for the rest of their lives. Ideally, people become 'expert' in managing the condition on a day-to-day basis. But they also need to know when and how to call on professionals for care and support. In these respects, diabetes is no different from a range of other chronic conditions. However, where diabetes differs from other conditions is that serious complications are likely to arise if diabetes is not well controlled, and these complications may have devastating consequences if they are not detected and treated early.

18. Evidence suggests that diabetes can have a markedly negative impact on quality of life, with individuals reporting concerns about restricted diet, work, family life, sex life and worries about the future. These negative effects tend to be more pronounced for those treated by insulin and for those who have developed complications of diabetes (Ref. 17). Coming to terms with the reality of living with diabetes can be very difficult, and psychological support can make a significant difference at this time.

---

1   Most recent total figure for acute and community trust spend from Trust Financial Returns for 1998/99 (Department of Health) was £21,294,137.

19. Care also needs to be tailored to the individual and their needs. Each patient has their own story of managing the condition and the care that they receive [BOX C]. This study considers how well patients are served by current diabetes services.

BOX C

Mrs A's story

Mrs A was 58 years old when she was diagnosed as having diabetes. She went to the doctor complaining of feeling dizzy and tired. On the second consultation, she mentioned feeling thirsty as well and was offered a urine test which suggested diabetes. At that time, she was told that she was only suffering 'mild' diabetes and encouraged to eat more healthily. She was a little confused about what this meant and carried on as usual, but eating fewer sweet things.

She was sent to the hospital after three months to confirm the diagnosis and receive a full review. This involved two bus journeys and she had to wait one and a half hours to be seen. The consultant examined her briefly and she was then seen by a specialist nurse who impressed on her the seriousness of the condition and possible complications that could develop if she didn't look after herself. This seemed at odds with what her GP had told her. She was told about foot care but didn't want to see a chiropodist as she felt there was nothing wrong with her feet. She saw a dietitian, but by that time she was very tired and didn't take in much of what was said. It took her over two hours to get home.

After that, Mrs A saw her GP and practice nurse every six months but continued going to the hospital once a year for an annual review. Her blood glucose control was fairly erratic and, after two years, she was prescribed insulin. This made her feel depressed and anxious about her ability to deal with the needles. She received a home visit initially from the diabetes specialist nurse, but then relied on support from her practice nurse. The old practice nurse, who knew Mrs A and her family, had left and the new nurse seemed to have too much to do. Mrs A relied on her husband to help her with the injections. She felt that she was failing to control her weight and missed the hospital appointment for her annual review as she didn't want to be 'told off' or asked about her insulin injections.

When she next saw the practice nurse for her six month appointment, her diabetes control was poor and she was found to have foot ulcers which needed urgent hospital treatment. She received care on a general medical ward and was not followed up by the hospital diabetes team. On discharge, she returned home to her husband and was seen again at her GP surgery some months later.

Source: Audit Commission

Patterns of care

20. Most people are diagnosed when they present with symptoms to their general practitioner (GP), sometimes by way of a district nurse or other professional like their local pharmacist [EXHIBIT 3]. Urine glucose levels are often measured initially, followed by further measurements of blood glucose levels to confirm the diagnosis. This is usually done by the GP, although 10 per cent of respondents in the Audit Commission survey of general practices referred all people with symptoms of diabetes to hospital without having confirmed the diagnosis themselves.

EXHIBIT 3

Patterns of care

There is considerable variation in patterns of routine care for people with diabetes.

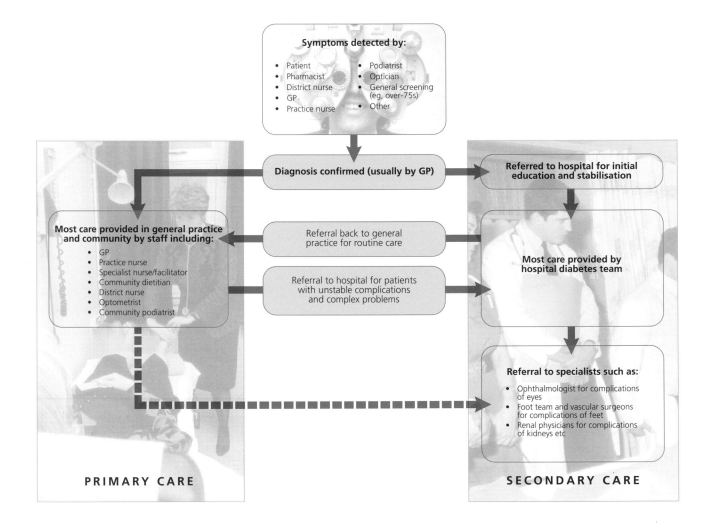

Source: Audit Commission

21. People with diabetes do not always have symptoms, in which case the diagnosis may be made during a routine medical check. For some patients, the lack of symptoms can mean that their diabetes is detected only when they begin to develop associated complications. The UK Prospective Diabetes Study (UKPDS) found that up to 50 per cent of people with Type 2 diabetes have complications on diagnosis (Ref. 16). In extreme cases, prosthetists have reported patients who were not aware that they had diabetes until they had to have a limb removed.[1] The National Screening Committee is now developing screening guidelines for diabetes, which should be published in 2001.

22. Once diagnosed, most Type 1 patients are seen by specialist diabetes teams, usually in hospitals, for initial treatment and follow-up care. The specialist multidisciplinary team should include physicians, specialist nurses, psychologists, podiatrists and dietitians – all with an interest and expertise in diabetes. The wider team includes associated specialists for particular complications. Children diagnosed with diabetes are routinely referred to hospital for their care. In the past, this was also true for all adults with diabetes. But patterns of care have changed and many Type 2 patients are now cared for entirely outside hospital, by a range of staff in general practice and the community (Exhibit 3). This trend was encouraged by changes to GP contracts and health promotion payments in 1990.

23. Since then, the role of primary care has been steadily increasing. The Government has given a commitment in recent policy statements to build on the 'increasingly important role of primary care in the NHS' (Ref. 18). A study in North West England in the early 1990s reported that 50 per cent of patients were managed wholly in primary care (Ref. 19) and this figure is probably far greater today. In 1997, the first national survey of the organisation of diabetes care was carried out (Ref. 20). In this study, GPs reported that they had a significant input to the diabetes care for 75 per cent of their diabetes patients. This suggests that it is now common for primary care teams to provide routine care for people with diabetes.

24. This trend was confirmed by a smaller Audit Commission survey of general practices **[EXHIBIT 4, overleaf]**, showing that most practices provided the majority of care for patients with Type 2 diabetes. But there is also considerable variation – more than one in five Type 2 patients in 10 per cent of the responding general practices were going to hospital for their routine care.

---

1   Personal communication from British Association of Prosthetists and Orthotists.

EXHIBIT 4

Where patients are treated

Practices reported different patterns of care, although the majority of Type 2 patients for these responding practices were managed in primary care.

Source: Audit Commission survey of general practices

Percentage of patients with diabetes at each practice

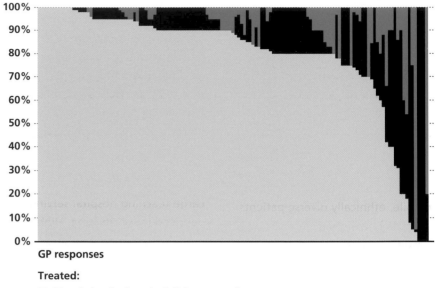

GP responses

Treated:

■ **Mostly by the hospital diabetes service**

■ **Jointly between the practice and the hospital**   ■ **Mostly in primary care**

25. The Audit Commission also carried out a survey of people with diabetes, using both hospital and general practice lists. The responses showed that some form of shared care – where patients are seen both by hospital and general practice staff for their routine diabetes support – was experienced by 28 per cent of respondents, but with substantial variation between districts (ranging from 12 to 52 per cent). The definition of shared care is unclear and can be interpreted in a variety of ways. To clarify this, the survey also asked whether respondents attended hospital for their annual review or health check. Not surprisingly, 87 per cent of the hospital sample attended hospital clinics for their annual review. But over half of respondents from GP lists in areas where primary care was not well developed were also attending hospital for annual review – as opposed to less than one-quarter from GP lists in other areas.

26. This suggests considerable variation across the country in where patients are seen, and by whom, and in the role of the hospital. This may be a reflection of patient preference, historic patterns of referral, the characteristics of the population and how well-developed hospital and primary care services are in particular areas [BOX D].

BOX D

A tale of two services

Some hospitals provide routine care for many diabetes patients while others focus more on education and support for staff working in different settings. The different roles of hospital diabetes teams may reflect differences in the populations that they serve – for instance, some areas have more mobile, ethnically diverse patients who may be higher users of hospital services. In addition, some areas have more developed primary care services that provide much basic patient care, freeing up hospital teams to focus on other activities. The Audit Commission's study visits showed a range of different models of care.

Trust A *(brief description)*

Trust in rural area with 4 per cent ethnic minority population and relatively well developed primary care. English is not the first language for 1 per cent of the population.

Trust Z *(brief description)*

Large teaching hospital serving deprived inner city area. Highly mobile population with large ethnic minority community (36 per cent of the catchment population), particularly from Afro-Caribbean communities. English is not the first language of 13 per cent of survey respondents.

Trust A appears to be more primary care oriented, with less than half the proportion of the trust catchment population on its

diabetes register compared to Trust Z. A survey of patients on primary care diabetes registers [TABLE 1] also showed that more respondents in the Trust Z than the Trust A population were usually seen at hospital, for all or part of their routine care.

Surveys of general practices in these areas confirm these findings. Practices in the Trust A area estimated that, on average (median), less than 10 per cent of their Type 2 patients received an annual review at the hospital, compared to 21-50 per cent in the Trust Z catchment area.

This brief sketch suggests that there are very different configuration of services and historic patterns of service use in different parts of the country.

TABLE 1

Routine patterns of diabetes care

Percentage of patients reporting they are usually seen in…

Patients sampled from	Hospital only	Primary care only	Care is shared
Trust A – primary care registers (n = 532)	15 per cent	73 per cent	12 per cent
Trust Z – primary care registers (n = 404)	23 per cent	41 per cent	36 per cent

Source: Audit Commission survey of people with diabetes[I]

I   P values in chi square tests confirm that differences between the two samples are significant and are unlikely to be due to chance.

27. The role of community trusts is also important, as they employ community podiatrists (sometimes also known as chiropodists) and dietitians, some specialist diabetes nurses, and other generic staff, such as district nurses, who are likely to be involved in the day-to-day care of people (particularly older people) with diabetes. A recent Audit Commission study of district nurses showed that up to 20 per cent of patients on district nurse caseloads at seven community trusts were related to diabetes (Ref. 21).

28. There is no clear evidence of what model of care is most effective for people with diabetes. But studies comparing standards of care in primary and secondary settings concluded that primary care can do as well as secondary care, where GPs have a special interest in diabetes, and where the care is well organised (Ref. 22). The configuration of diabetes services is considered in more detail in the last chapter of this report.

Evidence on diabetes

29. A number of landmark research studies have been concluded in the last ten years which make it an exciting time to review diabetes services [BOX E]. While the evidence on effectiveness is clear, with the exception of eye screening and particular elements of treatment, such as blood pressure control (Ref. 23), the cost-effectiveness of diabetes services has not been demonstrated. However, few professionals in the field doubt that effective prevention, management and early detection of problems is cost-effective in the long run.

BOX E

Sources of evidence on diabetes care

Recent research evidence has shown conclusively that good care can make a difference to long-term outcomes for people with diabetes.

Diabetes Control and Complications Trial (DCCT) (1993) (Ref. 24)

A US study which clearly demonstrated the benefit of improved glycaemic control in reducing the complications of Type 1 diabetes.

United Kingdom Prospective Diabetes Study (UKPDS) (1998)

(Ref. 1) (Ref. 16) (Ref. 25)

A major longitudinal study of people newly diagnosed with Type 2 diabetes which demonstrated the benefits of early diagnosis and intensive treatment. It showed clearly the progressive nature of the condition and highlighted the importance of blood pressure control and other risk factors as well as glycaemic levels, in reducing the complications of Type 2 diabetes.

Evidence on effectiveness – joint royal colleges initiative (1999) (Ref. 5)

The NHS Centre for Reviews and Dissemination produced an *Effective Healthcare Bulletin* in August 1999. This covered the complications of diabetes, reviewing evidence on screening for retinopathy and the management of foot ulcers. This work was part of a collaborative programme involving the Royal College of General Practitioners, the British Diabetic Association, the Royal College of Physicians and the Royal College of Nursing. This information will be used to develop evidence-based guidelines for health professionals in the diabetes field.

Source: Audit Commission

30. The findings may be summarised according to four main stages of care [TABLE 2]. At each stage, steps can be taken to prevent, delay or minimise the progression of the condition and to maximise the individual's quality of life.

TABLE 2

Diabetes – evidence on what works

At each stage, the research evidence tells us what can be done to improve outcomes for people with diabetes.

Key stages	Evidence
Prevention	
Maximising healthy lifestyles in the general population is likely to reduce the number of people with diabetes overall.	Control of obesity may prevent 50 per cent of new cases of Type 2 diabetes (Ref. 26).
Early detection	
Early diagnosis and treatment can reduce the risks of serious complications.	Up to half of all people with Type 2 diabetes already have complications on diagnosis (Ref. 16), which could have been prevented or treated if diabetes had been detected earlier.
Structured programmes of care and self-management	
Good education and support is essential to cope with diabetes and improve long-term outcomes by helping people to maintain optimum blood glucose and blood pressure levels.	Better blood glucose control reduces the risk of eye disease by one-quarter and of early kidney damage by one-third (Ref. 16). Blood pressure control has also been shown to reduce the risk of strokes and deaths from long-term complications by one-third (Ref. 25).
Surveillance and early detection of complications	
Regular checks of eyes, feet and other tests can ensure early detection of complications. Timely referrals and interventions can then minimise the effects of complications.	Eye screening and treatment can reduce the risk of severe visual loss or blindness among people with diabetes to less than half (Ref. 5). Foot protection and education programmes can reduce the rate of amputations by two-thirds (Ref. 5). Early laser treatment for eyes can also prevent up to 60 per cent of new cases of diabetic blindness (Ref. 25).

Source: Audit Commission

Structure of report

31. This report looks at current services and considers how well patients are being served at the four stages of diabetes care [**EXHIBIT 5**]. Chapter 2 examines the early stages of disease and the ways in which commissioning bodies – health authorities and, increasingly, primary care groups (PCGs) and local health groups (LHGs) – can target those at risk. It also looks at the commissioners' role in assessing the health needs of their communities, monitoring the quality of care, and planning services for the future.

32. Chapter 3 considers how care is delivered for people once they have been diagnosed with diabetes, focusing mainly on hospital services. It looks at the support and education provided for people with diabetes, the systems that trusts have in place to ensure good diabetic control, and effective surveillance and treatment of complications.

EXHIBIT 5

Four stages of diabetes care

This report examines the four stages of diabetes care at which effective interventions can make a difference.

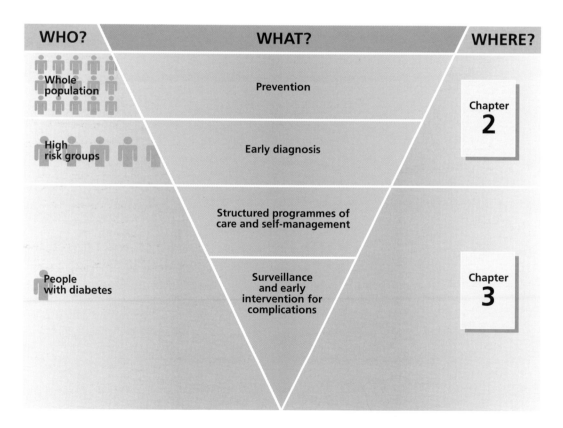

Source: Audit Commission

33. The final chapter discusses the challenges that face diabetes services now and in the future. It considers what needs to be done, in the light of rising demand on services, to ensure that people with diabetes are given the support and services that they need to live their lives to the full.

34. The research methods for this study are described in Appendix 1. The research was guided and supported by an expert advisory group, members of which are listed in Appendix 2. The report is accompanied by a programme of local audits of acute trusts in England and Wales in 2000. The local audits of hospital services, which form part of this study, complement other important initiatives that have been established in recent years to improve standards of diabetes care (Appendix 3).

Summary

...few professionals in the field doubt that effective prevention, management and early detection of problems is cost-effective in the long run

35. Diabetes is a major health problem:
- It causes substantial mortality and morbidity – some of it preventable.
- The large and increasing numbers of people with diabetes and increasingly intensive treatment regimes point to a substantial increase in the diabetes workload in the future.
- Significant NHS resources are spent on caring for people with diabetes – this will rise with increased workload.
- Clinical research has helped to confirm the features of services that are associated with good outcomes and provides a firm evidence base for the recommendations in this study.

36. The challenges facing diabetes services are to:
- help patients to develop skills to manage the condition effectively themselves and find an acceptable balance between diabetic control and preferred lifestyle;
- minimise the social and financial cost to society of the condition by effective treatment and early detection and management of complications; and
- provide an accessible and co-ordinated service for people with diabetes, combining a wide range of staff working in different sectors.

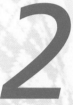

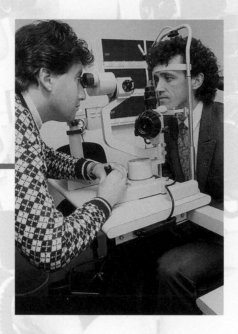

Planning Services

Diabetes services are often poorly co-ordinated and
fragmented. Those planning services often lack basic
information and few are monitoring the quality of care or
developing strategies to raise awareness or improve access to
services for high-risk groups. But some places have really
made a difference through outreach work, facilitators,
guidelines and training staff across sectors.

Introduction

37. The first step in developing first-rate care for people with diabetes is to understand the health needs of the population. There are important issues to be faced [BOX F], and the challenge lies in improving prevention through the promotion of healthy lifestyles, increasing rates of detection by raising awareness among health professionals and groups known to be at high risk, and ensuring the provision of services that meet the needs of the population.

38. These important activities are the responsibility of all those professionals who deliver diabetes care in hospitals and the community, as well as health authorities which have a strategic role in shaping services. In addition to health authorities, PCGs and LHGs now have an increasing role to play in these areas. There is also now much more focus on joint planning across health sectors and between health and social care agencies. The development of health improvement programmes and plans indicates the new spirit of partnership across sectors. The voluntary sector and individual users of services are also more involved in planning services, and the advent of groups such as Local Diabetes Services Advisory Groups (LDSAGs) have encouraged more lay participation in the development and monitoring of services. LDSAGs normally report to health authorities and should be present in every district, bringing together a range of health professionals from primary and secondary care sectors, as well as people with diabetes (Refs. 27 and 28).

BOX F

Key issues in planning services for people with diabetes include:

- The incidence and prevalence of diabetes is rising.
- The incidence of the most common form of diabetes, Type 2, can be reduced by preventive health strategies.
- Many people with Type 2 diabetes remain undiagnosed.
- As a result, up to 50 per cent of people have established complications at diagnosis.
- Complications develop in some people with diabetes because they are not receiving the education, treatment and monitoring that they need.

- Some groups, such as older people, those in residential care, people from ethnic minority communities and others may be at particular risk of inadequate monitoring and late diagnosis.

In addition:

- Many specialist services based in acute trusts are finding it difficult to manage ever-increasing workloads.
- Services are often fragmented, with unclear lines of responsibility across different sectors.

- Information needed to plan and monitor services and their outcomes is usually inadequate and often absent.
- Health professionals delivering services in community settings do not always have the training or support that they need.
- There is a growing emphasis on partnership with users and the importance of individually tailored care, but this is often overlooked by those planning services.

Source: Audit Commission

39. The themes covered in this chapter include:

- prevention and early detection of diabetes;
- information and monitoring quality;
- resource allocation;
- access to services;
- co-ordination of care; and
- changes in primary care.

Prevention and early detection of diabetes

40. Health authorities, PCGs and LHGs all have responsibility for primary prevention and raising awareness of diabetes in the general population. There are clear indicators that the incidence of Type 2 diabetes could be reduced by lifestyle changes in the broader community. Commissioning bodies should, therefore, be promoting healthy lifestyles including sensible eating habits, avoidance of smoking and the benefits of physical activity. These lifestyle changes are important for everyone, including people who have diabetes.

41. Of particular importance is the role of obesity. It has been estimated that reduced levels of obesity could prevent as many as 50 per cent of new cases of Type 2 diabetes (Ref. 26). But there has been a marked increase in obesity in the last two decades. The proportion of the adult male population that is obese rose from 6 per cent to 17 per cent and, for women, from 8 per cent to 20 per cent during the period 1980 to 1997 (Ref. 29). Effective strategies to limit obesity in the general population are likely to have benefits in reducing the overall demand for diabetes care.

...the incidence of Type 2 diabetes could be reduced by lifestyle changes in the broader community

42. As well as general primary prevention, commissioning bodies have an important public health role in raising diabetes awareness so that people recognise symptoms and present earlier. This could be done through schools, workplaces, social clubs, religious groups and other forums. Health authorities appear to be doing little to target people who are not only at greater risk of developing diabetes, but who may also find health education material less accessible. But some districts are making real attempts to meet this challenge [CASE STUDY 1].

43. The diagnosis and classification of diabetes has been subject to some debate recently, with revised criteria published recently by the World Health Organisation resulting in a lowered threshold for diagnosis (Ref. 9). At a local level, there is often uncertainty about the basis for diagnosis and the tests used. Many people are diagnosed with diabetes through routine clinics (such as those for the over-75s in general practice), or through contact with district nurses and others. Given the large number of people presenting without symptoms, some already with complications that could have been avoided, some practices have developed proactive measures to test people at risk of developing diabetes. These include factors such as age, ethnicity, family history of diabetes and obesity. There is great variation in approach at present and some places have developed local screening policies to ensure consistent practice for the communities that they serve. But 31 per cent of respondents in the Audit Commission survey of general practices had no local policy of screening for diabetes.

CASE STUDY 1

Health action zone to improve diabetes services

Health action zones (HAZs) are deprived areas that receive Government funding to tackle inequalities in health and to improve working across organisational boundaries between health and social services.

Bradford Health Authority has received HAZ funding to help establish an equitable diabetes service across the district, and to strengthen services to cope with increasing demands. The authority and practitioners already benefit from a comprehensive district-wide diabetes register to which 90 per cent of practices currently supply data which is used for audit and feedback.

The service will be based on an intermediate care model consisting of

- GP mini clinics providing comprehensive routine care for people with diabetes;
- satellite clinics for patients with more complicated diabetes and insulin dependent patients, run by GPs, diabetes specialist nurses and trained (diploma level) practice nurses, supported by a consultant and dietitians and podiatrists;

- hospital service for patients with major complications, new Type 1s, pregnant women and children; and
- a training programme for GPs and practice nurses that is provided locally and which must be completed by staff who wish to specialise in the diabetes service.

Developments aiming to improve detection, information and education include:

- a pilot project to identify non-diagnosed people, aged over 20 years in the South Asian population and over 40 years in the Caucasian population;
- joint working with the Benefits Agency to set up information points for people with diabetes about entitlement to benefits;
- working with health promotion staff undertaking patient education in the South Asian community;
- education programme for schools using a CD ROM and a website to encourage healthy lifestyles and awareness among children.

Resources have been put into the staff needed to ensure success including:

- a diabetes co-ordinator whose role is to make sure that plans are implemented;
- extra diabetes specialist nurses, podiatrists and dietitians;
- funding to sponsor a distance learning course for nursing home staff to improve care of residents with diabetes;
- a link person to work with the South Asian community in Bradford; and
- events to raise awareness in the general population.

Key features include:

- a service which is planned in response to local needs;
- a better educated general population;
- standardised care across the district, which dovetails with the health improvement programme to improve the quality of diabetes care; and
- a more equitable service in terms of accessibility, which offers patients greater choice and enables secondary care providers to provide specialist care.

Source: Audit Commission based on data from Bradford Health Authority

44. There is continued debate about the cost-effectiveness of systematic screening of populations for diabetes and policy on this issue is expected from the National Screening Committee in 2001. Those planning services should await the results of this national screening policy and, in the meantime, should be taking active steps to raise awareness among local health professionals and high-risk groups on the benefits of early diagnosis.

Information and monitoring quality

45. To ensure high quality services for people with diabetes, now and in the future, commissioning bodies need to:

- give diabetes high priority;
- carry out a needs assessment and review of diabetes and associated services in their area;
- establish a high quality, population-based diabetes register to provide information about patterns of care, processes and outcomes, and provide the evidence for service monitoring;
- monitor outcomes of diabetes care, both clinical and psychological, using established standards such as those set down in the St Vincent declaration (Appendix 3);
- plan services on the basis of current and projected need, particularly taking account of rising demand for care; and
- work with all providers of services and patients to meet these aims, using channels such as Local Diabetes Services Advisory Groups.

46. An Audit Commission survey of 26 health authorities showed that few had met these requirements [EXHIBIT 6]. However, it is encouraging that almost one-half of respondents had given priority to diabetes in joint planning arrangements, such as health improvement programmes (HIMPs) and, in Wales, health improvement plans (HIPs). Given the importance of diabetes, and the rising numbers, every district should feature diabetes in its planning process.

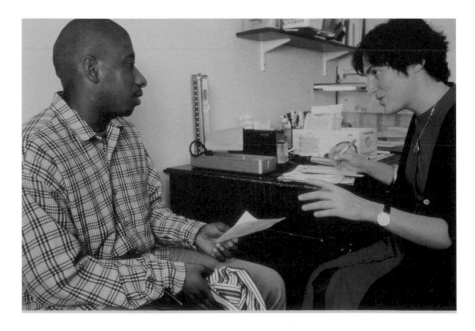

EXHIBIT 6

Survey of health authorities

Health authorities lack basic information to plan and monitor diabetes services.

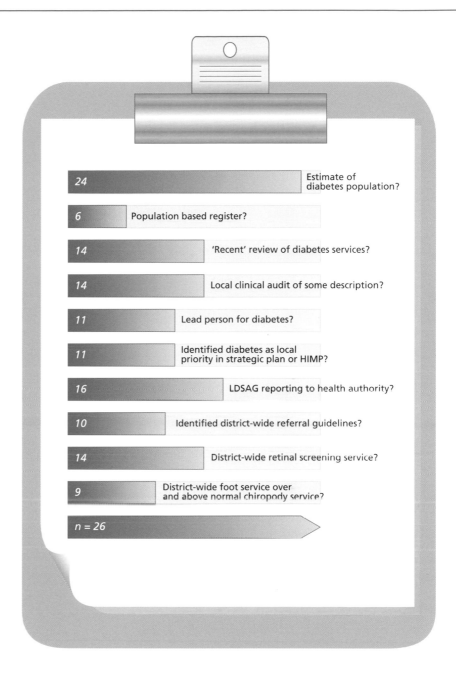

24	Estimate of diabetes population?
6	Population based register?
14	'Recent' review of diabetes services?
14	Local clinical audit of some description?
11	Lead person for diabetes?
11	Identified diabetes as local priority in strategic plan or HIMP?
16	LDSAG reporting to health authority?
10	Identified district-wide referral guidelines?
14	District-wide retinal screening service?
9	District-wide foot service over and above normal chiropody service?

n = 26

Source: Audit Commission survey of health authorities

Information

47. A recent Government paper has identified a 'menu' of useful clinical outcome indicators on diabetes for health authorities and others (Ref. 30). But the ability of health authorities to collect such data is often hampered by the lack of district-wide registers [**CASE STUDY 2**] or other system to monitor the health of people with diabetes. These should cover all people with diabetes, no matter where care is received, and should collect a minimum data set for diabetes care. Registers, with their mixture of process and outcome data, can play an invaluable part in supporting clinical governance and quality improvement programmes across a population. They are also useful in organising district-wide retinal screening programmes, with call and re-call facilities across populations.

CASE STUDY 2

Diabetes registers

Population-based information systems, such as registers, are essential for planning and monitoring diabetes services and can be used as part of a quality improvement programme.

South Tees Acute Hospitals NHS Trust has a long-established diabetes register, based at the diabetes centre at Middlesborough General Hospital. Although it is located at the acute trust, the register also covers patients who are managed in primary care. A diabetes specialist nurse is employed on a part-time basis specifically to facilitate this link with primary care and, where necessary, to collect information from practices for the register and ensure that it is accurate and up to date.

The register has been developed locally and can be changed to respond to the needs of the service and current developments.

Key features include:

- accurate data which can be used to audit the service provided by the trust;

- increasing coverage of the register in primary care for audit purposes;

- the use of a standard form for collecting clinical information which has improved record-keeping and helps with continuity of care;

- a perception of increasing accuracy of primary care based data and wider 'ownership' of data; and

- stronger links with primary care through visits by the specialist diabetes nurse which has helped to strengthen continued professional development as well as improve record-keeping.

Source: Audit Commission

...many health authorities were unable to collect data on outcomes of diabetes care

48. The St Vincent declaration (see Appendix 3) set clear targets for diabetes care more than ten years ago.[I] But only four out of 26 health authorities surveyed had set local targets in line with the St Vincent declaration. Information systems were found to be highly variable in the extent to which they provide good population-based data, and many health authorities were unable to collect data on outcomes of diabetes care. These deficiencies will be highlighted when the National Service Framework on diabetes is published in 2001, which is likely to require more active monitoring by commissioners of services, trusts and practices.

49. Considerable efforts are being made to tackle the absence of good information and it is hoped that many of the current problems will be addressed as the NHS Executive Information for Health strategy is implemented over the next five years. In addition, the British Diabetic Association (BDA) is developing the UK Diabetes Information Audit and Benchmarking Service (UKDIABS) which aims to improve the standards of information for diabetes care and provide a common database with information on patient interventions and outcomes (although records to date are far from complete).[II]

Monitoring quality

50. Commissioning bodies need information to assure themselves of the quality of services, and clinical governance requirements will reinforce that need. But the Audit Commission survey of health authorities showed that only half had carried out a recent review or audit of diabetes services. It appears that many health authorities know little about the care being delivered or its quality. However, in some places, health authorities have worked together with local primary care audit groups to monitor diabetes services in primary care [**CASE STUDY 3, overleaf**].

51. The smaller size of PCGs and LHGs (discussed more fully at the end of this chapter) and the emphasis on peer review, mean that quality assurance in primary care may be more feasible than for health authorities [**CASE STUDY 4, overleaf**]. Some PCGs are developing initiatives, such as identifying lead or specialist GPs on diabetes. The new clinical governance arrangements provide opportunities for PCGs and others to set priorities for reviewing the quality of certain services. In a recent Audit Commission survey (Ref. 33), one in five PCGs had identified diabetes as one of their top four priority areas for reviewing clinical governance arrangements in primary care. This would include arrangements for audit, education, record-keeping and information systems, as well as processes for patient care.

I   As well as the high-level targets, detailed guidance was produced for those planning and delivering diabetes care (Ref. 31).

II   There is also a programme, DIABQoL+, which provides validated measures of psychological outcomes and processes against which services can measure changes in quality of life (Ref. 32).

CASE STUDY 3

Health authority review of diabetes care

The health authority has a key role in monitoring the health of the population and providing an overview of diabetes services across all health sectors.

Dorset Health Authority has developed a comprehensive clinical audit of diabetes care across the district. It covers 97 practices and around 13,300 patients. The audit has been running since 1993/94, so that trends in healthcare coverage can be monitored. Data collected includes prevalence of condition plus coverage of tests such as foot examination and blood glucose levels. Information covers all patients who are diagnosed with diabetes and are registered with a general practice, *regardless of the source of care*. This means that, importantly, the database covers patients treated mainly in general practice as well as those receiving care from hospital.

The audit is administered by a Clinical Outcomes and Audit Group (COAG), at one remove from the health authority but with full-time staff funded by the health authority.

COAG provides results for each individual practice, including comparative data between practices. However, individual reports remain confidential and are not available to the health authority. An anonymised aggregate report is produced for public consumption. Results are discussed and disseminated through local medical networks, as well as by publishing the report. COAG is also responsible for producing guidelines on issues such as standards and training needs for practice nurses.

In 1998/99, COAG produced an audit of outcomes to complement the established audit of processes. Forty per cent of Dorset practices signed up to this audit. This is part of a move towards measuring outcomes as the gold standard, and as a necessary prerequisite for improving quality in primary and secondary care.

Key features include:

- comprehensive data on annual review coverage for district-wide diabetic population;
- coverage of patients who are treated in both primary and secondary care;
- practices that can review individual performance through confidential reports; and
- comparative data that provides information on intra-district variation in patient care, reviewing processes and outcomes.

CASE STUDY 4

Assessing quality through primary care

PCGs, LHGs and health authorities are experimenting with ways of monitoring the quality of diabetes care.

In **Croydon**, diabetes has been identified as a priority for clinical governance arrangements. Parchmore Medical Centre and the public health department of Croydon Health Authority worked together to provide some baseline information. Data was collected on routine management of Type 2 patients at Parchmore Medical Centre. This was used to develop some indicators, which were discussed at a study afternoon for GPs within that PCG. Indicators included items such as proportion of patients whose HbA1c levels had been measured. Each practice was encouraged to set its own targets for clinical governance, which were realistic.

Key features include:

- involving practices in setting achievable local targets;
- using one practice to illustrate process to others; and
- using a study day to support GPs in setting standards.

At the **Royal United Hospital, Bath** the trust has identified lead GPs for each of the five PCGs in its patch. The aim is to get PCGs signed up to care plans to develop minimum standards for primary care in their patch as part of their commitment to improving patient care and satisfying clinical governance requirements. The diabetes links in each PCG meet regularly, providing a forum to discuss standards of care, referral criteria and new developments in diabetes care.

Key features include:

- developing diabetes specialism in general practice;
- using PCGs to disseminate information to their individual practices, to ensure consistency of care across a trust catchment, and to allow audit of outcomes; and
- training and professional development opportunity for GPs.

52. Health authorities, PCGs, LHGs and others also need to be planning ahead for the dramatic increase in numbers of people with diabetes. But there is little evidence that this is happening. Bodies such as Local Diabetes Services Advisory Groups (LDSAGs) can be very helpful in bringing together staff across sectors and disciplines, as well as patients, to consider ways of developing and reconfiguring services. However, 10 out of 26 authorities surveyed had no LDSAG reporting to them. The last chapter of this report discusses in more detail the growing pressure on services and suggests options for meeting future needs.

Resource allocation

It is not easy at present to identify the resources that are devoted to diabetes care...

53. It is not easy at present to identify the resources that are devoted to diabetes care, so it is difficult to assess the adequacy of funding for a particular service, and more or less impossible to make meaningful comparisons between districts and trusts. In hospitals, diabetes services are usually funded from the general medicine budget, and cannot be identified separately. Many staff, such as doctors and dietitians, are not dedicated to diabetes care, and it is difficult to quantify their input. Staffing levels vary and some posts are funded by 'soft monies' such as research grants or voluntary monies. This makes it difficult to compare resources across sites – in addition, some specialist diabetes teams are funded wholly by the acute hospital, while others are part funded by community trusts and health authorities (for instance, diabetes facilitators).

54. The lack of clarity about resources for diabetes care has in itself been a problem for those planning and providing services. This is particularly evident in the funding of retinal screening programmes, which currently receive support from a variety of sources. Some health authorities have dedicated resources to establishing district-wide programmes, but in other places it is left to trusts and general practices to find the resources.

55. In primary care, diabetes services are funded as part of general medical services, through the Chronic Disease Management Programme (CDMP). This is a basic payment to general practices of approximately £400 for every GP who provides a diabetes service, currently received by 98 per cent of GPs in the Audit Commission survey of general practices. The budget-holders for this programme tend to be health authorities, but at present there are only basic requirements to qualify for payment, including a register of diabetes patients, rather than specific guidance on expected standards of care. The Audit Commission survey of health authorities showed that only half had undertaken any audit of this programme.

56. Explicit acknowledgement of the level of care provided by a practice, via audit of the CDMP, would allow payments for such services to be related to activity and quality. The NHS Executive should review the CDMP, considering targeting payment so that practices providing comprehensive diabetes care are rewarded appropriately, and ensure that staff who provide services are suitably trained. In the meantime, commissioning bodies might consider ways of adding value to the present system. For instance, one health authority (See Case Study 23, p105) has involved one of its leading diabetes centres in the CDMP payment, linking it to programmes of training and quality assurance for general practices that have been set up by the diabetes centre.

57. More explicit links between resources and measures of quality are likely to feature more heavily in the next decade, in the light of the National Service Framework on diabetes and arrangements for clinical governance. Health authorities and trusts therefore need to consider ways of identifying and managing resources to ensure greater accountability for the services provided.

Access to services

58. Those planning services have a responsibility to make sure that the populations that they serve receive good quality care. This includes the physical access to services and providing support and advice to people with diabetes at the times when they need it. Commissioners also need to understand the nature of their population and the problems of access experienced by particular individuals and groups.

Access for people from ethnic minority communities

59. People from ethnic minority communities, for example, may not get the services that they need because of differences in language, literacy and culture [BOX G]. Many problems experienced by people from ethnic minorities are common to all people with diabetes, but given the high prevalence of diabetes in some ethnic groups, it is especially important that services respond to their needs. The condition is three to six times more common in South Asian people, and two to three times more common in Afro-Caribbean people, than in the Caucasian population (Ref. 3).

BOX G

Mr Ps story

Mr P is an Asian man in his late 40s, working in a small business. He complained of feeling tired and thirsty, but did not go to the doctor's for some time. His father and several of his older brothers had diabetes, but Mr P saw this as an 'old man's' condition and didn't think that he was affected.

When he did go to his GP, he was told that he had diabetes and should go to the hospital for confirmation. This made him feel very down, as he felt that he had failed as head of the household and would not be able to provide for his family. His knowledge of diabetes included his father being very ill in his last years with kidney disease and failing eyesight. He also felt ashamed at being upset and did not want to share his fears with a young female GP.

He was told about changes to his eating habits, but his wife (who managed the household diet) did not speak English and was not contacted by the diabetes team, so no particular changes were made. In any case, the information he received related to foods that he was not familiar with, like Cornflakes and tuna fish. It did not include dietary advice that was relevant to Asian families. One concern he had early on was what to do during Ramadan, when he was not meant to take food or medicines.

Continued overleaf

BOX G (continued)

He went to the hospital three months later and was very embarrassed to be weighed in the public waiting area by a nurse. He could speak English passably well, but did not read it. He was given leaflets from the BDA and the local hospital, but did not say that he could not read this material. The doctor examined him but spoke very fast and Mr P did not understand what he meant by 'retinal examination' and 'podiatry'. He was told how to monitor his blood glucose, but did not like the idea of drawing blood. When he went home, he gave the meter and strips to his wife to look after and she put them in a drawer.

In the meantime, his wider family became aware of his condition. His nephew, who had been looking after his own father with diabetes, got hold of leaflets in Urdu from the British Diabetic Association and talked them through with Mr P. His mosque also organised a 'diabetes awareness day' with the local health authority and he was able to talk to other people in his community with diabetes, including people of his own age.

At his next visit to the GP, he went with his nephew and the GP arranged with the hospital for an interpreter to be present for his structured review at the hospital. For this review, he went with his wife, and the presence of an interpreter meant that they could both have a meaningful dialogue with the doctor, dietitian and the specialist nurse. He was still reluctant to discuss his anxieties about the condition, but felt more in control of his diabetes and that he was not alone.

60. The increased prevalence in ethnic minority communities relates to Type 2 diabetes, probably due to a combination of genetic predisposition and lifestyle factors. In addition, blood glucose and blood pressure control is known to be more erratic, and diabetes-associated mortality higher in these groups (Ref. 34). Knowledge about diabetes and risk factors tend to be poorer, too, in these groups, as demonstrated by published evidence (Ref. 35) and Audit Commission findings [TABLE 3].

61. While some research has been done into the characteristics of different Asian groups, there is little in the literature on black African and Caribbean people with diabetes. But while much of the evidence presented here relates to Asian groups, differences in cultural beliefs, attitudes and dietary customs also exist in black African and Caribbean communities, and these are extremely relevant to the management of diabetes.

TABLE 3

Patients' understanding of diabetes

Patients from ethnic minority communities reported poorer levels of understanding about key features of diabetes [Note 1]

Percentage of respondents who reported [Note 2]	Ethnic minority n = 202	Other groups n = 1,176
Not feeling confident that good control could prevent long term complications	13	6
Understanding little or nothing about the effects of being ill on diabetes control	48	24
Understanding little or nothing about taking exercise	21	9
Understanding little or nothing about diet and how it affects health	16	6
Understanding little or nothing about smoking and its effects on health	13	5
Understanding little or nothing about what to expect if blood glucose drops too low	29	19

Note 1: P values in chi square tests confirm that differences between the two samples are significant and are unlikely to be due to chance.
Note 2: Results from six of ten questions asked about patient understanding of diabetes.

Source: Audit Commission survey of people with diabetes

62. Some of the key issues affecting ethnic minority groups include:

- Wide variation in literacy rates according to age, sex and ethnic origin. While some groups may speak one language, they may read in another. This affects the nature of written and other patient information that is needed (Ref. 36).

- Cultural variations in attitudes to ill health and disease and healthy diet and lifestyles. This includes attitudes to body image and to the treatment of ill health, including the use of alternative remedies. Dietary education in particular needs to be culturally sensitive (Ref. 37).

- Potential stigma attached to people with diabetes in some groups (Ref. 38).

- Conflict between religious practices, such as fasting, and usual recommended approaches to diabetic control. This requires more imaginative approaches to accommodating diabetes care to the patient's own lifestyle.

I do not read English or Urdu. Therefore my care information should be in another format, like an audio tape in mother tongue language. There should always be an interpreter available at the clinic.

Audit Commission survey of people with diabetes

Services can tackle these issues in different ways [**BOX H, overleaf**].

BOX H

A good diabetes service for people from ethnic minority communities will:

- have information on the ethnic make-up of its population and target resources accordingly;

- be aware of languages spoken, literacy rates, dietary practices, alternative remedies and religious practices;

- have sought out views on the service provided;

- have appointed staff to reflect the ethnic population, where possible, and train all staff on cultural and religious aspects of diabetes care;

- have an accessible and well used interpreting service;

- provide translations of basic literature, such as the BDA leaflet *What to Expect* (Ref. 39) and appropriate audio tapes;

- have a policy for detecting diabetes in high risk groups;

- give advice on matters such as diet which is sensitive to cultural differences [Note 1];

- monitor outcomes by ethnic group; and

- be making attempts to increase awareness of diabetes among high risk groups.

Note 1: Professionals can seek advice from the British Dietetic Association, which has a specialist multicultural nutrition group.

Source: Audit Commission

People from ethnic minority communities may not get the services that they need because of differences in language, literacy and culture

63. As a first step, those planning and delivering diabetes services need to know about the ethnic composition of their patients. This information is necessary to identify the needs for language services among their service users. In areas where there are highly diverse populations, or large numbers of people from particular ethnic groups, some trusts have developed comprehensive translation services. They may employ link workers and advocates to assist with the consultation. In some parts of the country, special attention has been given to make services more accessible to people from ethnic minority communities [CASE STUDY 5]. Other examples include Leicester, where the Nutrition and Dietetic Service run an Asian study day for all new staff and students to raise cultural awareness. Commissioners should be aware of such initiatives and should encourage similar approaches in areas where access to services for minority groups is poor.

CASE STUDY 5

Access for ethnic minority patients with diabetes

At Derbyshire Royal Infirmary, efforts have been made to identify and meet the needs of the ethnically diverse population. This has been done in collaboration with the community trust, and jointly funded posts have been developed for this purpose.

The service consists of:

- a consultant-led outreach clinic with interpreting services present;

- staff who are conversant in local languages and aware of cultural issues, particularly in relation to diet; and

- targeted patient education for people from the Asian population, and those who do not speak or read English. These have evolved to meet the expressed needs of the population, for example, single sex education sessions.

Key features include:

- accessible services for people from the Asian community;

- a tailored education programme to respond to the needs of the population; and

- a perception of improved attendance rates among patients from the Asian community (although this has not been evaluated).

Source: Audit Commission study sites

64. It is more difficult to arrange such services in areas with very small numbers of people from ethnic minorities. But it is essential that these people, too, can participate fully in clinical consultations and benefit from written (and other) information. This is particularly true in primary care settings which are geographically dispersed. In order to tackle this issue, some diabetes professionals have established networks with others around the country, to share information and expertise relating to providing accessible care for particular ethnic groups.

Access to advice

I wish there was someone I could speak to when I don't feel well in the weekend.

65. Since self-management is such an important feature of diabetes, patients need to have access to support and advice as the need arises [Ref. 39]. The Audit Commission patient survey showed substantial variation in whom patients would contact for advice about their diabetes

...20 per cent of patients said that they did not know who they could contact about their diabetes at night or at weekends

during working hours, depending on where they routinely receive their diabetes care [TABLE 4]. But the most common source of help was staff in general practice.

66. The survey also asked about access to advice out of hours. It is worrying to note that 20 per cent of patients said that they did not know who they could contact about their diabetes at night or at weekends. This emphasises the need for good communication between professionals and the need to inform patients about the services available to them.

I have nobody to contact after hours and sometimes feel very alone with this.

67. There are different approaches to providing out-of-hours services: for instance, some trusts visited for this study provided patients with the number of a mobile phone, carried by a member of staff on a rota basis. Others, such as Derbyshire Royal Infirmary, had established a 'duty' system whereby diabetes specialist nurses provided cover for a dedicated telephone line. Their time was protected from other clinical duties while on duty, so that immediate advice was available each morning. Arrangements for out-of-hours support was an area that was often under-developed due to lack of resources. Seven out of the nine trusts visited by the Audit Commission did not have formal arrangements for patients to contact staff at weekends. Access to out-of-hours support and advice is an area that those commissioning services should review.

TABLE 4

Access to help and advice

Who would patients contact with questions about their diabetes during working hours?

Patients sampled from...	Percentage of patients reporting whom they would contact [Note 1]				
	GP	Nurse at general practice	Hospital doctor	Specialist nurse at hospital	Don't know who to contact
Hospital registers [n = 460]	32	11	21	32	4
Rural district – primary care registers [n = 532]	51	33	5	8	3
Urban district – primary care registers [n = 404]	49	22	12	11	5

Note 1: Respondents could select more than one option.

Source: Audit Commission survey of people with diabetes

Physical access

68. The physical aspects of access are also important and those planning services need to consider how to make services easy to reach. For example, a rural area with poor transport links might develop a network of satellite clinics to provide specialist support to a dispersed population [CASE STUDY 6]. Others have tackled specific pockets of poor access, providing clinics in cottage hospital settings. Where access to a specific service, such as retinal screening, has been identified as a problem, domiciliary visits have been established for housebound patients, or a mobile screening service established.

CASE STUDY 6

Diabetes specialist nurses covering geographically isolated areas

In the **Bath** catchment area (serving a population of 550,000), four diabetes specialist nurses are employed by the local community trusts. They cover a patch that is rural and not well-served by public transport. The nurses work on a locality basis and have their own caseload of patients. Patients come to them by open referral – mainly from GPs, practice nurses and district nurses, some from the diabetes specialist team and secondary care, but also by patients themselves.

The nurses run specialist diabetes clinics in different parts of the locality and each clinic provides patient education and support for changes of treatment and lifestyle. Each nurse will see about a hundred patients a month, with a mixture of booked appointments and drop-in service. Specialist nurses also train link nurses at community hospitals, to improve inpatient care for patients on geriatric and other wards. Another key part of the service is telephone contact with patients.

An important part of the specialist nurse role is to provide support and training for staff in primary care. Each locality covers about 24 practices and the specialist nurse sits in on some of these diabetes clinics and provides telephone advice for practice nurses and GPs. As part of a training programme, the nurse convenes Diabetes Special Interest Group meetings, held at different GP surgeries in the district, which attract between 30-50 GPs, practice nurses and district nurses. The impact of providing structured training for practice nurses is currently being evaluated as part of a research project.

Key features include:

*   specialist nurse-run clinics that relieve some of the hospital workload and provide specialist care near to patients;

*   continuity of support for practice nurses and GPs;

*   improved patient education across primary and secondary care; and

*   liaison between acute trusts, community trusts and general practice.

69. Patients with foot problems may not be physically mobile, so staff need to let them and their carers know in advance about parking arrangements and access for wheelchair users. And many older people with diabetes have impaired vision, so written information and letters need to be prepared in large type. These practical issues concerning access can make a real difference to patients.

Co-ordination of care

I sometimes find that the advice given at the hospital clinic differs from that given by the diabetes nurse attached to the hospital. This again sometimes differs from advice given by my doctor's practice diabetes nurse. It is clear that different people do things in different ways but when advice is not consistent this can be problematic.

70. Commissioners also have an important role in ensuring that services are well co-ordinated. Patients sometimes report lack of co-ordination between the professionals caring for them, and confusing and inconsistent information [TABLE 5]. It is particularly difficult where professionals are working in different organisations or geographical areas, because records and case-notes may be conflicting or incomplete.

TABLE 5

Co-ordination and communication in diabetes care

Proportion of respondents agreeing that...

Sometimes doctors and nurses don't seem to have all the information they need about me.	18%
I don't understand who all the people are who are treating me.	11%
I often have to give the same information about my diabetes to different people at the clinic.	24%

Source: Audit Commission survey of people with diabetes (n=1,075)

71. There is a real problem too in the isolation experienced by staff delivering care to people with diabetes in the community. A recent study showed that 34 per cent of primary care diabetes clinics were run by practice nurses alone (Ref. 20). Although this survey showed that in 88 per cent of practices, one or more of the practice nurses had attended a diabetes training course within the last three years, the course duration was variable. Practice nurses are key members of the diabetes team, but may not find it easy to obtain peer support and keep abreast of developments in diabetes. Community nursing staff may experience similar isolation. While half of community trusts surveyed for this study employ specialist diabetes nurses – on average, two per trust – more than one-quarter employ only one whole time equivalent (WTE) post or less. Those planning diabetes services need to make special efforts to support staff in the community by arranging training and meetings to share knowledge among professionals in the same field.

Two district nurses said my tablets would make me lose weight, but the diabetes nurse said different, said the tablets make you fat. It is this kind of information which makes you not want to bother. You don't know which advice to believe.

72. Other staff involved in diabetes care include community podiatrists, dietitians, specialist diabetes nurses and district nurses. A recent national survey of dietitians found that only half said that there was a dietitian whose job it was to co-ordinate dietetic services for people with diabetes in their area (Ref. 40).

73. Health authorities and other commissioning bodies can improve co-ordination in a number of ways [BOX I]. Professional development, training, clinical audit and teambuilding across disciplines are discussed in more detail in the next chapter.

BOX I

Approaches to co-ordinating diabetes care

Different measures can be used to make care more integrated for the patient including:

- facilitators and liaison nurses/other staff;
- Local Diabetes Services Advisory Groups;
- shared record systems and use of electronic patient records;
- developing multidisciplinary and multi-sector training programmes;
- multidisciplinary clinical audit; and
- developing, implementing and monitoring guidelines.

74. Some initiatives that are funded by health authorities such as diabetes facilitators [CASE STUDY 7] appear to be effective in providing consistency of care across different settings.

CASE STUDY 7

Co-ordinating diabetes care through facilitators

Diabetes facilitators can play a crucial role in co-ordinating care across sectors.

Lambeth, Southwark & Lewisham Health Authority set up the *Diabetes Resource Team* – two diabetes facilitator posts funded by the health authority and managed by the community trust. These posts were occupied by specialist nurses, who carried no patient caseload so that they could concentrate on supporting and training GPs and practice nurses and link back to the four main acute trusts. Their link with trusts is mainly on issues that impact on primary and secondary care, to work towards ensuring that patients are seen in the most appropriate setting. Links with PCGs are being developed.

The facilitators visited 163 practices for baseline assessment of diabetes services. The assessment focused on the ability of practices to provide adequate facilities for people with diabetes; maintain effective registers; introduce proper systems for re-call and develop protocols for referral. Following these initial visits, practices were ranked roughly to target those practices most in need of support and development.

The Team also provided training for staff in primary care. This included two five-day courses for practice nurses each year and a Diabetes Forum for general practitioners held four times a year, which was approved for Postgraduate Education Allowance (PGEA). The Health Authority also funded a popular 'in-reach' scheme for GPs to shadow hospital diabetes staff for 12 sessions. There were also sponsored lunchtime meetings for practice nurses and district nurses held in rotation across the patch.

Key features include:

- practical support for primary care staff, particularly practice nurses running diabetes clinics, thus improving standards in primary care;
- cohesion across sectors and disciplines; and
- comprehensive training for a wide range of primary health staff.

Source: Audit Commission

75. It is also important to co-ordinate care and training of staff across a district within each discipline. It is sometimes helpful to identify responsibility for a particular care group across a geographical area.[1] This has been done for the care of the elderly in some places, who are an important group in diabetes care [CASE STUDY 8].

---

[1] Staff such as district nurses caring for older people tend not to be dedicated to diabetes care, although this makes up a significant part of their workload. The lack of a disease-specific focus may be entirely appropriate given the problems of co-morbidity, especially in older patients. For example, two-thirds of the patients on district nursing caseloads who receive a diabetes care package were also receiving care for another condition (Ref. 21).

CASE STUDY 8

Co-ordinating diabetes care of elderly people

A significant proportion of diabetic patients are elderly. Their diabetes may be compounded by a number of other complaints and some may also be confused and in need of special attention.

The **Royal Hallamshire Hospital in Sheffield** offers a once-weekly clinic for elderly people with diabetes who have cognitive or physical disabilities, poor diabetes control, or who are treated with insulin. The clinic is run by a consultant physician/geriatrician with a special interest in diabetes, and a diabetes specialist nurse with links to specialist community nursing staff for home visits.

The consultant geriatrician has also arranged funding for a research nurse post to review the care of elderly people with diabetes. This post is filled by an experienced diabetes specialist nurse who is trained in the assessment of diabetes, cognitive function, activities of daily living, self-care abilities and quality of life, and provides one-to-one advice on managing diabetes to patients, families, carers and other healthcare professionals. The research post also fulfils an education and training role, giving input into diabetes nursing courses and study days.

Work has been done to identify training needs for a range of staff. The specialist nurse has carried out a survey of nursing and residential homes in the Sheffield area to assess the prevalence of diabetes and uptake of community services, such as diet advice, foot care and eye screening services. In addition, the geriatrician and specialist nurse, along with a GP and practice nurse, form the elderly subsection of the Local Diabetes Services Advisory Group. Their main remit is to review community services for people in care homes, and to pursue permanent funding for a designated diabetes specialist nurse for the elderly.

Key features include:

- a designated clinic combining geriatrician and diabetes specialist nurse expertise;

- a combined clinical/research post which contributes to the development of co-ordinated diabetes services for the elderly, as well as carrying out clinical and nursing research in the speciality; and

- provision of training and support for staff such as district nurses, practice nurses and residential home carers/staff.

...guidelines were often incomplete, out of date, or not used

76. Patient-held records, which are successful in antenatal care, have been developed with varying degrees of success for diabetes care (see Case Study 15, p73). In the long run, electronic patient records should help to ensure that all professionals have the necessary information to ensure well co-ordinated clinical care. This technology is not yet widely available, but some trusts are using the same principles to circulate brief, standard format output from local IT systems. This appears to ease communication between hospital doctors, specialist diabetes nurses and general practitioners. In the future, such technology should embrace all the professionals who care for people with diabetes.

Developing guidelines

77. Developing guidelines with input from a range of staff across sectors is a good way of improving the consistency of care for patients. They can be used locally to indicate which kinds of patients will benefit from the care of specialist teams and those who could normally be managed by primary care staff.

78. Guidelines should be based on the best available evidence and should be tailored to take account of local circumstances. Successful guidelines have input from a wide range of staff to ensure ownership [CASE STUDY 9]. The process of developing guidelines is often a good teambuilding exercise in itself.

79. Despite the potential benefits, the Audit Commission survey of general practices showed that 41 per cent do not have written guidelines for referring patients to hospital diabetes services [EXHIBIT 7, overleaf]. Only 19 per cent of practices were using hospital or district-wide guidelines and even fewer had developed joint guidelines with the local hospital. At hospitals visited by the Audit Commission, guidelines were often incomplete, out of date, or not used.

CASE STUDY 9

Local guidelines and protocols

A well-run diabetes service normally develops clear guidelines so that responsibilities and practice are consistent throughout.

At **Poole Hospital**, guidelines have been drawn up for assessing the feet of people with diabetes. The guidelines are used by GPs, practice nurses, district nurses and other staff. They were developed by a range of staff, including podiatrists, vascular surgeons and diabetologists. Guidelines are as simple as possible and include clear diagrams of feet and indications of what to expect. Criteria are used to categorise patients into low, medium or high risk for neuropathy and vascular disease, based on clinical indications. The guidelines give action plans for different risk groups, suggesting routes of referral – for instance, high risk vascular patients should be referred directly to the vascular surgeon.

CASE STUDY 9 (continued)

Key features include:

- a method of increasing the appropriateness of referrals (ie avoiding late referrals for urgent foot problems);

- a tool for educating staff in general practice and community on diabetes care; and

- clear and simple guidelines that could be used by a wide range of staff.

At **Dorset Health Authority**, guidelines have been developed for practice nurses. Three different guidelines have been drawn up, depending on the extent of nurse involvement with diabetes care. This ranges from a minimal role, where the nurse is merely screening patients before a GP consultation, through to a maximum role, where the nurse is running a diabetes clinic and working with the GP to make decisions about the care and treatment of individual patients. For each level, details are given of clinical responsibilities (for instance, at the maximum level, working with a GP to adjust insulin doses) and educational responsibilities (for instance, teaching the patient about foot care, at the medium level). There are also recommendations for nurse education and training at each level.

Key features include:

- clear standards for practice nurses, outlining practical tasks and responsibilities;

- standards tailored for different levels of involvement; and

- focus on education and training needs at different levels.

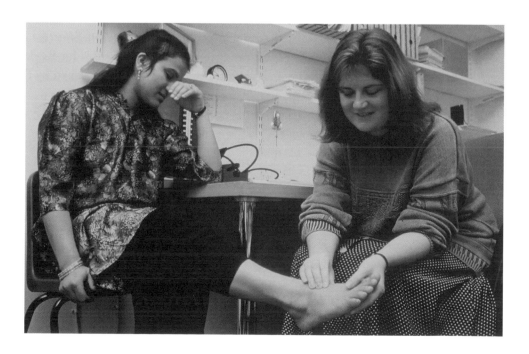

86. Perhaps the biggest change will come when some PCGs/LHGs become providers of community services as PCTs. For diabetes care, this may mean employing community specialist diabetes nurses, podiatrists, dietitians and other community nursing staff. There may be opportunities to provide more integrated services for people with diabetes – a 'seamless service' – by appointing liaison staff to act as co-ordinators of diabetes care over a manageable population base. At present, some places are currently experimenting with liaison posts for certain client groups that are funded jointly by health authorities and community trusts. There may also be greater scope for interdisciplinary training and teambuilding events for all staff who are involved in the care of people with diabetes, working in community and primary care settings.

87. The emergence of PCTs may provide an incentive for practices to shift care for people with diabetes from the acute to community sector. At present, this is speculation only – the impact of these organisational changes in primary care is difficult to predict. But it is likely that the reshaping of primary care will have a direct impact on patterns of diabetes services in years to come.

CASE STUDY 10

PCGs as commissioners of diabetes care

PCGs and LHGs will be starting to commission services and develop specifications for hospital care for patients in their catchment.

South Kensington, Chelsea and Westminster Primary Care Group is introducing a *quality bond* with its local hospital for a number of services, including diabetes. Instead of a block service level agreement for diabetes, the PCG is agreeing a fixed sum and then setting conditions for the additional monies. These conditions have been developed by PCG primary care staff working with the local public health consultant from the health authority. As a first step, the standards are based on process measures, such as the proportion of diabetic patients who have had their blood pressure taken. The aim is that, in time, the standards might include clinical outcome measures, such as the proportion of diabetic patients whose blood pressure reading falls within set limits.

Key features include:

- primary care staff setting standards for hospital care;
- commissioning to include quality measures; and
- improved information about the patients' health status and treatment.

Summary

Diabetes services are often not well-planned and few places are making provision for future increases in demands

88. This chapter discusses the present role of health authorities, and the emerging role of PCGs/LHGs, in planning and monitoring diabetes services. Key points include:

Prevention and early detection of diabetes

- There needs to be more multi-agency effort to raise awareness of diabetes and to develop health promotion programmes, particularly on obesity. There is currently confusion about how to increase detection rates of diabetes, with almost one-third of general practices having no local guidelines on screening – national policy from the National Screening Committee in 2001 will be very welcome.

Information and monitoring quality

- Health authorities often lack basic information to monitor the health of people with diabetes – only 6 out of the 26 surveyed had some form of district register. Little priority has been given to diabetes, with just under half of authorities not having undertaken a recent review of services.

- There was little evidence of forward planning by health authorities, despite the dramatic increases in patient numbers expected in the next decade. Planning and service development would need to involve staff and patients across all sectors, but 10 out of 26 authorities had no formal Local Diabetes Services Advisory Group reporting to them.

Resource allocation

- It is difficult to identify current resources for diabetes services, and this lack of clarity may cause problems of accountability. One concern is the current system of payment for general practitioners' work on diabetes, which is not linked to activity and quality, and should be reviewed.

Access to services

- Access to services for people from ethnic minorities is often poor. A patient survey showed poorer levels of understanding about diabetes among respondents from ethnic minority communities – for instance, half did not understand the impact of an illness like flu on their diabetes, compared to one-quarter of non-ethnic respondents.

- People with diabetes need access to support and advice at all times, but one-fifth of patients surveyed didn't know whom to contact outside working hours. Seven out of the nine hospitals visited had no formal arrangements for out-of-hours cover.

Co-ordination of care

- People with diabetes may see many different staff in different settings, but care is often poorly co-ordinated. For instance, one-quarter reported having to give the same information to different professionals. Some places have better co-ordinated services, and have used facilitators and multidisciplinary training events to achieve this result.

- Guidelines developed with input from a range of staff can be useful to provide more consistent care. But 41 per cent of practices reported no written guidelines for referral – despite evidence (for instance, with foot problems) of late referrals.

Changes in primary care

- The development of PCGs and LHGs provides real opportunities for better monitoring and planning of local diabetes services. Exciting initiatives include the identification by one trust of lead GPs in each PCG to make care more consistent across its patch. The development of PCTs in the future may provide more opportunities for better co-ordinated care for chronic conditions, such as diabetes.

89. Successful planning needs good information and partnership between professionals, agencies and users of services. This chapter has indicated that diabetes services are often not well planned and few places are making provision for future increases in demands. The next chapter looks in more detail at the care which is delivered and considers the ways in which services can be improved to meet the needs of people with diabetes.

RECOMMENDATIONS

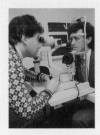

2 Planning Services

Health authorities and PCGs/LHGs need to:

Improve the prevention and early detection of diabetes

1 include a section on diabetes in local health improvement programmes and plans. This should cover actions to educate their population about risk factors and raise awareness of diabetes, particularly in high risk groups. [Paragraph 42]

Improve information for planning and quality control

2 establish and maintain population-based information systems, such as registers, to monitor the health of people with diabetes. These should have up-to-date information on health outcomes and investigations, and be linked to call-recall systems for structured reviews. [47]

3 work with clinical audit colleagues to review diabetes services in the community and feed back results to local practices. District-wide audits across primary and secondary care are helpful for developing relationships across sectors, as well as joint monitoring. [50]

4 monitor processes and outcomes, including a range of clinical and psychological measures, and support change where necessary. Those planning services should consider clinical governance arrangements for diabetes as a priority. [51]

5 use information from the register and other demographic data to make estimates about future demands on services and work with providers and patients to plan against these estimates. [52]

Improve management of resources

6 work with trusts and PCGs/LHGs to identify staffing and monies dedicated to diabetes care, ensuring proper systems for managing resources. [57]

Improve access to services

7 review patient satisfaction with current services and identify populations at need, particularly ethnic minority groups, and review current use of services. Where problems of access are identified for ethnic minority patients, initiatives such as interpreting and translation facilities should be considered with service providers. [63]

8 review arrangements for people with diabetes to receive support and advice out of hours. [67] Also identify areas where physical access is poor, and work with service providers to develop outreach services and other solutions. [68]

RECOMMENDATIONS

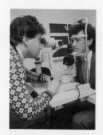

2 Planning Services

9   ensure the provision of comprehensive district-wide retinal screening programmes, in line with the recommendations of the National Screening Committee when they are published in 2001. [68]

Co-ordinate diabetes services across sectors

10   establish and support a Local Diabetes Services Advisory Group with multidisciplinary clinical and lay input to identify areas for improvement and promote the integration of services, from a patient perspective. [73]

11   work with diabetes teams in acute trusts to facilitate ongoing training for GPs, practice nurses and community staff. [75]

12   facilitate the development of clinical guidelines, including guidance on the kinds of patients who would benefit from the care of specialist teams and those who could normally be managed in primary care, given adequate facilities, training and support. [77]

The NHS Executive and National Assembly for Wales need to:

Improve the prevention and early detection of diabetes

13   promote widely the findings of the National Screening Committee when it reports on diabetes. [44]

Improve information for planning and quality control

14   ensure that the Information for Health strategy addresses some of the concerns about poor information for diabetes services identified in this report. [49]

Review resource allocation

15   review the monies available to GPs, including the Chronic Disease Management Programme payments, to identify opportunities for more effective targeting of payment to the activity and quality of diabetes services provided. [56]

16   review resources associated with diabetes across sectors and clarify current funding arrangements in the forthcoming National Service Framework. [57]

Improve the co-ordination of services across sectors

17   develop, implement and evaluate evidence-based multi-professional guidelines on the management of people with diabetes. Guidance on best care should form part of the National Service Framework in 2001. [80]

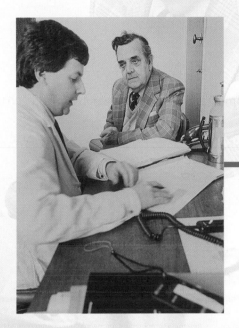

3

Delivering Effective Care

Self-management is the key to good diabetes care and patient
education should be at the heart of any service. But many
trusts are not providing comprehensive, lifelong education for
their patients. Regular health checks are also crucial, but there
are important gaps in reviews to detect early complications,
especially of eyes and feet, and often poor co-ordination
between the diabetes team and associated specialties. More
can be done through improved record-keeping, initiatives
such as joint clinics, and investment in professional education
and development.

Introduction

90. The last chapter considered the foundations and structure that a service needs to minimise the incidence of diabetes, detect it early, and to provide planned, co-ordinated care. This chapter examines the nature and content of these services, focusing largely (but not exclusively) on the work of hospital specialist teams, which formed the bulk of fieldwork for this study and is the subject of a programme of local audits throughout the year 2000.

91. From the point of diagnosis, people with diabetes need structured programmes of care with a strong focus on education and self-management. Diabetes is a lifelong condition, and self-management is the key to minimising its effects. Diabetes services also need systematic programmes to check the health of people with diabetes and to detect, at an early stage, complications that are amenable to treatment.

92. This chapter covers:

- *Supporting self-management*
  The ways in which services can support people with diabetes to manage the condition effectively themselves. This includes sections on patient education, psychological support and satisfaction with services.

- *Surveillance and early intervention for complications*
  The ways in which services can provide routine and systematic checks for people with diabetes. It also considers the way in which services respond to complications, once detected, with particular emphasis on complications affecting the eyes and feet.

- *Care of special patient groups*
  The needs of special groups of patients, including inpatients with diabetes, children and pregnant women and how well services address these.

- *Improving quality*
  The support needed for staff to deliver high quality services for people with diabetes. This includes information, co-ordination across sectors, training and professional development. Examples are given of services that have invested in their staff to improve the quality of care for people with diabetes.

Supporting self-management

93. The importance of self-management across a range of health problems was stressed in recent Government policy (Ref. 42). Motivating and supporting people with diabetes to look after themselves is a priority task for any diabetes team. A key element for effective self-management is patient education.

Patient education

I did not realise how serious diabetes was at first. Perhaps I might have taken it more seriously if I knew then what I know now.

94. Good quality patient education has a number of key components [BOX J].

BOX J

Content of patient education for people with diabetes

Patient education should enable people with diabetes to:

- begin to come to terms with diabetes, understanding that this is a lifelong condition that they can learn to control and adapt their lifestyle to diabetes with the help of health professionals;

- know the basics of the condition and the complications that it can cause and when to access more information as they need it;

- understand the importance of controlling blood glucose levels (and how this is done), blood pressure and other risk factors;

- understand the importance of regular clinic attendance (in whatever setting) and the need for good foot care, eye checks and other areas where serious complications can be prevented or delayed;

- understand the need for healthy eating and exercise and the ways in which lifestyle, particularly diet, can be modified to maximise wellbeing;

- [where relevant] have the skills and confidence to manage insulin, including injection techniques and action in case of emergency (hypoglycaemia);

- understand the effect of illnesses on diabetes and what action they need to take when they are ill;

- understand the services, who does what, and points of contact for further advice and support as well as understanding what situations require immediate contact with health professionals;

- know about patient groups and how to get in touch with other people with diabetes; and

- understand that diabetes management is a continuous process and treatment can be adjusted in the light of changes in a person's life and lifestyle.

Source: Audit Commission

95. But a patient survey carried out by the Audit Commission showed that 67 per cent of respondents (n=1,390) reported no contact in the last 12 months for education and support and 40 per cent reported no contact on dietary advice. The survey also revealed significant gaps in patient knowledge and confidence in managing the condition. While the great majority of patients reported that it was worthwhile to control their diabetes, and believed that they understood the increased risks associated with the condition, a small minority were not at all confident that good control prevents complications.

I have no idea whatsoever why I do daily blood-checks...I have not the remotest idea what I am keeping the record for.

96. There were also deficits in understanding, with more than one in four respondents saying they understood nothing, or very little, about the effects of being ill on their diabetes, and one in five reporting that they did not know what to expect if their blood glucose dropped too low. As discussed in the previous chapter, these results were even more pronounced for respondents from ethnic minority groups. These findings highlight the importance of patient education as an ongoing activity throughout the lives of people with diabetes. Diabetes services need to make sure that the patient education that they provide satisfies a number of criteria [BOX K].

BOX K

Some features of high quality diabetes patient education

Patient education should offer:

- a structured programme for people who have been newly diagnosed with diabetes, including a written curriculum (including psychological as well as medical need);

- multidisciplinary delivery (including podiatrists and dietitians);

- varied modes of delivery, including both group and one-to-one sessions;

- access for newly diagnosed and established patients;

- continuous assessment and a programme for established patients according to individual needs;

- access to patients regardless of who delivers care; and

- built-in evaluation via assessment of each patient's knowledge and self-care.

---

97. Arrangements for patient education were variable across the trusts visited for this study. To some extent this was due to different levels of resources. Specialist diabetes nurses were key to the development of sound patient education programmes and all trusts visited for this study provided one-to-one sessions with specialist nurses for newly diagnosed patients. But in other ways, trusts were failing to deliver comprehensive structured programmes of education. In particular:

- four out of nine did not have a structured programme of education with a written curriculum;

- only four out of nine sites routinely involved podiatrists, despite the importance of preventative foot care. However, dietitians were routinely involved in patient education at eight out of the nine hospitals visited.

- only two out of the nine sites had any routine follow-up for established patients with diabetes; and

- only one hospital had taken steps to evaluate the education that patients received.

98. The lack of emphasis on evaluation is disappointing. It is possible to evaluate the effectiveness of different methods of patient education – ranging from group sessions, through videos, to intensive counselling – by testing outcomes such as knowledge, psychological wellbeing or actual biomedical markers of diabetes control. The BDA recently commissioned a literature review of education and psychosocial interventions for people with diabetes (Ref. 43). The authors found that the largest effects were associated with longer programmes that employed behavioural and psychological approaches to patient participation, rather than offering information alone. Indeed, increasing knowledge alone had little effect on targeted self-care behaviours. The 57 trials and 7 meta-analyses reviewed demonstrated methodological weaknesses; better-designed evaluation studies are needed. A further review in the form of an *Effective Healthcare Bulletin* is in preparation, which should provide more guidance to staff. In the meantime, services should build on what is known, and avoid relying on didactic methods of information-giving alone.

My attitude has always been 'it ain't going to beat me' and I believe that the most important care is education in all aspects of the disease…I have been insulin-dependent for 43 years and can still do 10 press-ups…It is not all doom and gloom!

99. Some trusts have made great strides in developing their patient education programmes [CASE STUDY 11]. At these trusts, patient education was seen as a specialist function of the hospital diabetes team serving the whole district, including patients who are managed mainly in primary care.

100. Some trusts have made great efforts to ensure that they tailor education programmes to the needs of individuals, including those people from ethnic minority communities. At Derbyshire Royal Infirmary, for example, specific sessions for Asian patients have been developed.

CASE STUDY 11

Patient education

Patients need effective education and support to help them to maintain healthy lifestyles and manage their diabetes.

Ipswich General Hospital puts patient education at the centre of diabetes care. All patients' visits to the diabetes centre should include an education component. For newly diagnosed patients, there is a structured programme of education led by a multidisciplinary team of staff. The programme includes one-to-one and group sessions. A range of tools is used, including an interactive patient education video with information about living with the condition. The diabetes centre evaluates the effectiveness of its programme of patient education by testing knowledge and understanding 'before and after' the patient begins the course. This was the only one of the nine sites visited by the study team to evaluate its approach to patient education.

Key features include:

- multidisciplinary approach to patient education;

- education incorporated into routine appointments with diabetes team; and

- patient education evaluated for effectiveness.

Poole Hospital offers a three-month structured programme of education for newly diagnosed Type 2 patients, which culminates in a consultation and review with a doctor. The first session covers basic information about diet, monitoring and diabetes and is open access – normally by referral from GPs. This is a group event, in a dedicated diabetes facility, with a chance for newly diagnosed patients and their family or friends to meet others in the same situation. The following session, about two weeks later, is by appointment. Each patient has their feet examined by a podiatrist and receives individual advice from a dietitian. At the third session, six weeks later, a diabetes specialist nurse explains the services and prepares the patients for long-term self-care.

Only after patients have been through this complete programme

are they seen by a consultant – about four weeks after the last education session. The doctor assesses the patients and about 60 per cent whose blood glucose levels are stabilising are referred back to their GPs for continued care. By the first appointment, the consultant knows which patients can effectively manage themselves (having changed their diet) and which patients need further help and treatment. Staff at the diabetes centre also provide training and support to GPs and practice nurses (the 'Diabetes Healthcare Club') and follow-up sessions for patients.

Key features include:

- structured programme of care with input from a number of health professionals and both group and individual sessions;

- opportunities for consultant to review impact of initial education after three months; and

- system for 'returning' patients to care in general practice.

Patient satisfaction

The initial diagnosis of my condition by my GP was quick and the care and attention I received at xxx Hospital, followed up subsequently at the diabetes centre, was nothing short of excellent. My rapid progress and control enabled me to modify my treatment from insulin down to tablets and now by diet alone. This must be attributed to the advice and care provided by all the medical staff concerned.

101. Many people with diabetes report quite high levels of general satisfaction with their care and recognise the commitment of the staff supporting them. However, surveys of people attending hospital diabetes clinics for this study identified the following common areas of concern:

- Not having enough information about, and opportunities to use new developments (24 per cent of 538 respondents at 9 study sites);

When I do attend the hospital, my consultant is always so overworked, she never has the time to talk about new things concerning diabetes.

- Waiting times (22 per cent of 665 respondents);

I am always seen 1-1fi hours after the time of appointment...when I attend the clinic, my blood pressure increases!

- Lack of opportunity to talk to other patients (19 per cent of 530 respondents); and

*Unless you are diabetic and have had problems, you will **never** know how a diabetic feels – lonely, fed-up and some days just wishing they were normal!*

- Lack of privacy in waiting areas (8 per cent of 657 respondents).

Some issues [concern people like me]...like being asked about your contraceptive choices as you queue for blood tests.

102. The Audit Commission's random survey of people with diabetes identified similar issues, when asked to highlight areas for improvement [EXHIBIT 8].

EXHIBIT 8

Aspects of care most in need of improvement

Concerns were particularly marked for patients in the samples from hospitals...

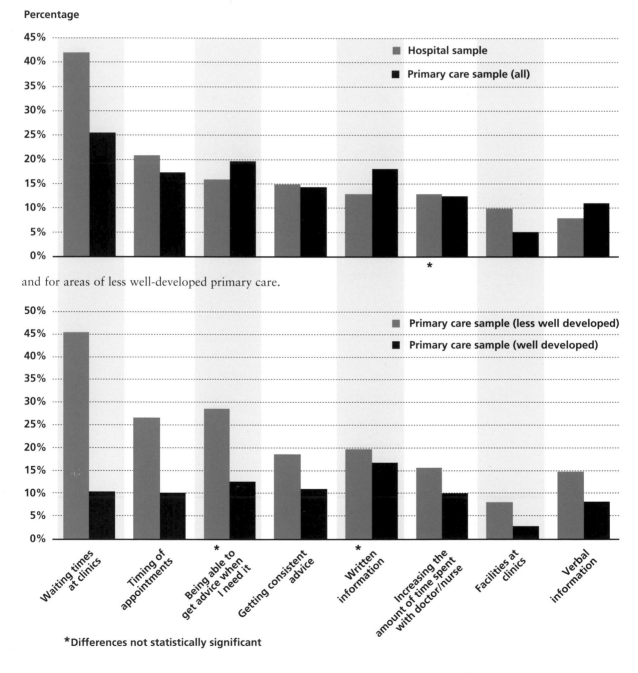

and for areas of less well-developed primary care.

*Differences not statistically significant

Note 1: Hospital sample [n=460]; primary care (well developed) [n=532]; primary care (less well-developed) [n=404].

Note 2: Chi square tests showed that all the differences were unlikely to be due to chance, except for those marked * where differences were not found to be significant.

Source: Audit Commission survey of patients

103. Some diabetes services have used patient satisfaction surveys to identify areas of weakness and to target resources on areas for improvement [CASE STUDY 12].

CASE STUDY 12

Using patient satisfaction tools to improve services

The Royal Sussex County Hospital, Brighton used a validated tool, the Diabetes Clinic Satisfaction Questionnaire, three times over a period of six years to measure satisfaction with its diabetes services.

Following the first period of data collection, interventions were designed to target three major sources of dissatisfaction: continuity of care, waiting times and privacy. Clinic staff took results to hospital management as evidence of areas of patient dissatisfaction, and requested additional funding to allow implementation of the interventions. The bid was successful. Doctor lists were modified to improve continuity, an extra session was included to reduce waiting times and walls were built around consulting areas to replace screens and improve privacy.

The first follow-up of the survey showed significant reductions in patient dissatisfaction in all three targeted areas. Where the survey had been used, clinicians were also able to predict more accurately patient concerns, suggesting that the process had improved health professionals' awareness of patient views. A recent follow-up data collection, five years on from the intervention, revealed that improvements had continued over time.

Key features include:

- use of validated tool to collect data systematically about areas of patient dissatisfaction;

- identifying and prioritising areas for action, with evidence to support bids for more resources;

- improved sensitivity to actual patient concerns by clinicians following use of structured survey; and

- follow-up work planned to measure the impact of interventions which were implemented after initial concerns were identified.

Source: (Ref. 44)

104. Another possible indicator of patient satisfaction is the rate of non-attendance at booked clinics. This averaged 20 per cent across the nine hospitals visited by the Audit Commission, but there was an almost four-fold variation between trusts [EXHIBIT 9]. A recent review of the literature on non-attendance in diabetes clinics underlined the importance of this problem, as these patients tend to have more risk factors and complications than those who attend. Evidence suggests different reasons for non-attendance (Ref. 45) from patient health beliefs to features of the organisation of services, but trusts need to make efforts to understand this better and take active steps to reduce it. One trust dramatically reduced non-attendance rates by requiring patients to reapply for appointments through their GP if they failed to attend without informing the clinic beforehand, although this caused unhappiness among some patients. It is clear that services need to take steps to maximise attendance – and, equally, that patients have responsibilities to make the best use of services that will help them to manage their condition.

I ask for help and the last doctor I saw told me if you don't follow the programme, don't waste our time. I didn't go back to the clinic.

105. Some trusts have adjusted clinics to improve service use – for example, providing early evening clinics for some groups of people, and single-sex clinics for others. Others run 'drop-in' or open access clinics where no appointment is needed. Services need to evaluate the impact of any changes that they make to identify the steps that are effective for different groups of patients.

EXHIBIT 9

Non-attendance rates at diabetes clinics

There was almost four-fold variation between trusts in non-attendance rates at clinics.

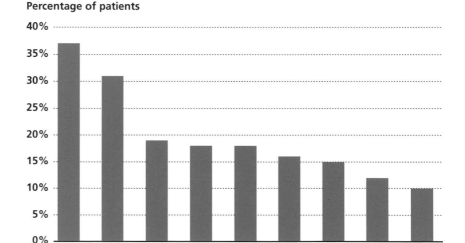

Percentage of patients

Study site

Source: Audit Commission clinic resource surveys

...it is important that [patients'] psychological and educational needs are treated as seriously as their medical needs

106. A common concern of patients is the length of waiting times for first consultant appointments, ranging from 4 to 14 weeks at the trusts visited. These waiting times suggest that many trusts are failing to comply even with minimal Patient Charter standards. But in areas where waiting times are high, some trusts have introduced interim appointments with a diabetes specialist nurse to ensure that the patient is not waiting too long before contact with an expert in diabetes care.

Psychological needs

I do feel I am a number and not a person with my own individual needs.

107. People with diabetes are more likely to suffer from clinical depression than those in the general population (Ref. 46) and services should make explicit provision for psychological support throughout the patient journey and should monitor psychological outcomes of care. Guidelines have been produced as part of the St Vincent initiative, indicating the steps services can take to improve psychological wellbeing for people with diabetes (Ref. 47). Some hospitals have recognised these needs (Ref. 48), but six out of the nine trusts visited failed to provide the services of a psychologist either to support patients directly, or to help professional staff to meet patients' psychological needs. Few sites routinely measured psychological outcomes or patient wellbeing.

It's important for me to have quick and direct contact with diabetes nurses, dietitians, doctors etc as this helps me to maintain good control of my diabetes... I also find that talking with fellow diabetics when attending clinic for appointment or for pre-arranged meetings through the diabetes unit helps me, as I know I am not alone.

108. Trusts can take active steps to support patients by facilitating the activities of patient groups (including group education sessions for newly diagnosed patients) and encouraging people with diabetes to become involved in local British Diabetic Association (BDA) groups. All staff providing care to people with diabetes need good counselling and listening skills, and should avoid blaming patients who fail to reach particular targets. Diabetes is a condition where individuals are largely responsible for the management of their own condition day to day. To achieve this, it is important that their psychological and educational needs are treated as seriously as their medical needs and become an integral part of care for everyone.

Routine surveillance

109. The BDA has set out clear guidelines on what patients should expect in the form of routine care (Ref. 39) and there is good consensus among professionals about minimum standards of care. These reflect research findings which demonstrate the cost-effectiveness of good blood glucose and blood pressure control in improving long-term outcomes and the importance of regular surveillance and treatment to minimise the effects of serious complications. This section provides an overview of how well services meet these standards.

Structured review

110. The structured review has become a cornerstone of good diabetes care, underlined in recent policy documents (Refs. 27, 28 and 49) and by the BDA. (Ref. 39). Systematic reviews can help to detect complications at an early stage, to highlight problems of diabetes control, and to identify people who are at risk of coronary heart disease and kidney failure. The evidence is not conclusive on the ideal frequency and modality (type of test) for different aspects of surveillance (Ref. 5), but there is good consensus on what should be included in a structured review [TABLE 5]. This is usually carried out every one to two years.

I would welcome a system where every person with this condition is called in at least once a year for a check-up. I am not a person who keeps running to my GP for minor worries, but I do feel alone.

During the course of the study it became evident that:

- some patients fall through the net and do not receive structured reviews at all;
- data and record-keeping on structured reviews can be poor, making audit difficult; and
- where data do exist, they show that surveillance can be incomplete or of poor quality.

111. Six of the nine hospitals visited for this study could not identify the proportion of their patients that had received complete structured reviews in the preceding 18 months. Of the three sites that did keep this information, estimates ranged from about one-third to three-quarters of patients receiving complete structured reviews. This may reflect poor record-keeping, rather than poor clinical care, as the Audit Commission user survey showed that 95 per cent of patients themselves reported having had some sort of annual check-up. Nevertheless, trusts should be able to monitor the care that they provide.

112. A sample of patient notes at each of the nine hospital sites showed variation in how well different parts of the review was recorded [TABLE 6]. For example, on average one in five patients reviewed had no record of a foot examination in the notes. There is also great variation from trust to trust, and practice to practice. In one trust, almost half of all patients had no record of a foot examination, and patients themselves are often unclear about what checks they have had. For example, 45 per cent of those responding to an Audit Commission survey reported either not having had, or not being aware of having had an HbA1c measurement (see glossary) to review their glycaemic control in the previous year. To make the processes of care clearer for patients, and to monitor progress, staff should develop explicit care plans for individuals, and allow people to agree the targets that they would like to aim for.

TABLE 6

Record of annual review items in medical notes

Some items are recorded far more frequently than others.

Element of annual review	Purpose	Frequency recorded
Weight	Obesity is a risk factor for diabetes. Weight control and healthy diet are important in diabetes control.	✔✔✔ (>90%)
Blood pressure	Raised blood pressure is a major risk factor for complications of diabetes, including coronary heart disease, stroke and kidney failure.	✔✔✔ (>90%)
Glycosylated haemoglobin (HbA1c*)	An indication of average blood glucose levels over the preceding 2-3 months.	✔✔✔ (>90%)
Fundi* examination	Observation of retina through dilated pupils to detect diabetic retinopathy*	✔✔ (75-90%)
Foot examination	Feet are examined to check for ischaemia* and neuropathy* which can cause ulceration.	✔✔ (75-90%)
Visual acuity	To identify deterioration in vision that may be indicative of diabetic retinopathy.	✔✔ (50-75%)
Serum cholesterol	Diabetes is a major risk factor for coronary heart disease.	✔✔ (50-75%)
Kidney function	Tests to detect early kidney disease, such as the presence of traces of albumin* in the urine.	✔✔ (50-75%)
Body mass index	An index of weight to height, considered a superior measure of obesity.	✔ (<50%)

Note 1: Definition of terms marked * given in the glossary.

Source: Audit Commission review of 270 casenotes at 9 study sites

I wish that I could have a regular check-up at the same place with the same people.

113. People with diabetes go to different settings for their structured review and some patients reported confusion over who was responsible for what and problems in continuity of care over time. Of patients sampled from primary care registers (with predominantly Type 2 diabetes), between one-quarter and one-half attended hospital for annual review, but used general practice services for their routine care. However, the majority of people with Type 1 diabetes attended hospital for their reviews.

114. The variations in proportions of patients attending hospital may reflect the resources available for full review in general practice [**EXHIBIT 10**]. For instance, less than one in three practices had routine input from a dietitian or podiatrist to their diabetes clinics. The different resources available to practices affect their ability to carry out full systematic assessments of patients with diabetes.

EXHIBIT 10

Facilities for diabetes care in general practice

Not all practices have the range of staff and resources to carry out full annual reviews on their premises.

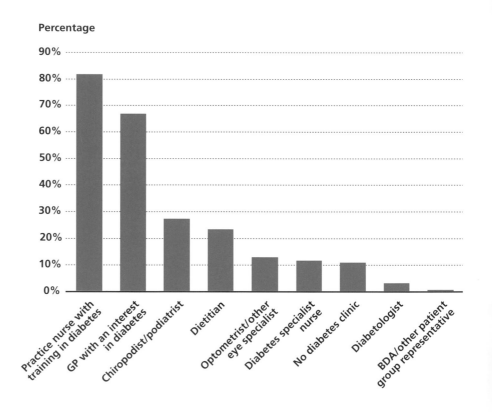

Source: Audit Commission survey of general practices

Without good organisational links [between specialties], serious delays in treatments can occur

115. Deficiencies in information on annual reviews is part of a wider problem of record-keeping in diabetes. The UKDIABS project (see Glossary) has been set up to improve the quality of routine information on diabetes care, including elements of the structured review. But not all health authorities have subscribed to this, and returns show incomplete data. For example, one of the responding sites had no recorded data on feet and eye checks, and only 25 per cent of patients had any record of cholesterol levels. Few centres were routinely measuring psychological processes and outcomes in patients, although tools are now available to help with this data collection (Ref. 32). It is clear that more effort needs to be made to collect and validate this sort of data.

Responding to complications

116. Effective preventative care can minimise the effects of diabetes, but services will always be needed to treat complications. It is crucial that the diabetes team has effective links with other specialties in the hospital that will treat patients for sight-threatening retinopathy, revascularisation procedures and managing end-stage chronic renal failure. Without good organisational links, serious delays in treatments can occur. The way in which diabetes teams can connect systematically with associated specialties is addressed more fully in the section on professional links at the end of this chapter.

117. Success in detecting complications at an early stage depends on a high level of awareness among both patients and professionals. Patients may not recognise complications, and so may delay seeking treatment. Similarly, professionals may fail to detect early complications which are amenable to treatment, particularly of the eyes and feet.

Complications affecting the eyes

118. A comprehensive district-wide retinal screening programme is an essential part of any effort to detect early complications of the eyes. The health authority's role in this programme was discussed briefly in the last chapter. Its importance was underlined in a recent bulletin which estimated that comprehensive screening and treatment for diabetic retinopathy could prevent about 260 new cases of blindness every year in the UK (Ref. 5). Screening can effectively be provided by trained and accredited optometrists (high-street opticians) or by retinal photographers in a variety of locations (Ref. 50). There should be a central register with a call and recall facility, proper training for staff and a system for checking the quality of the process – but these features are only present in some districts [CASE STUDY 13, overleaf]. At present, there is no general agreement on a common standard against which to measure the sensitivity and specificity of eye screening. This should be addressed when the National Screening Committee issues guidance on screening for diabetic retinopathy, which will inform the National Service Framework in 2001.

CASE STUDY 13

Diabetic retinopathy screening

The **Bro Taf Diabetic Retinopathy Screening Service** is a community-based, district-wide service that has been funded by the health authority since April 1998. The service aims to provide annual fundal (see glossary) photography for people with diabetes – approximately 18,000 – in the Bro Taf district. Currently 90 per cent of these patients are on the screening database, and the aim is to include as many patients as possible in the screening programme. A steering group reports to the health authority twice a year and reviews performance.

The service uses state of the art digital cameras and systems in two mobile screening units that are staffed by a retinal photographer and a healthcare assistant. The units travel to locations within the health authority and patients are sent appointments for screening at the site that is most convenient to them. Opportunities are taken, through patient groups and local meetings, to raise awareness among patients about the screening service.

The service employs a manager, a part-time secretary, and two full-time readers as well as the co-ordinators, photographers and healthcare assistants. In many ways the success of the programme is dependent on four locality co-ordinators who are based at the four local hospitals. They are responsible for obtaining lists of patients with diabetes from general practices and keeping a central database, with a call/recall system, up to date. They liaise with local practitioners about the screening service and monitor non-attendance.

At screening, visual acuity is checked, pupils are dilated and at least two photographs of the retina taken. All images are saved to laptop computers and later transferred to a system which is accessed by two trained graders for primary grading. The grading system is a three-tier one carried out respectively by primary graders, clinicians and ophthalmologists. Telemedicine links are being developed to enable remote access for ophthalmologists and GPs. There are quality assurance procedures built into every step of the process.

Reports are generated for the patient's GP and/or diabetologist, who are responsible for giving patients results. The screening service may refer directly to an ophthalmologist if patients have sight-threatening retinopathy.

Key features include:

- state-of-the-art screening near to patients;
- a well-supported programme, including locality co-ordinators at local hospitals; and
- good quality assurance in a three-tier checking system.

EXHIBIT 11

Features of retinal screening programmes

Not all places had comprehensive retinal screening programmes with the necessary measures to assure quality.

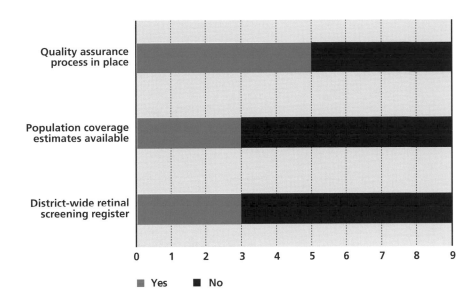

Source: Audit Commission study sites

119. Study site visits showed a range of approaches to retinal screening [EXHIBIT 11], with many places lacking data on coverage. In the three districts where estimates of coverage were possible, these ranged from one-half to three-quarters of the target population.

120. Also, local information on cases of blindness is frequently poor. Given its value in monitoring outcomes of diabetes services, it is important that this information be improved. One study site had conducted a retrospective review of all registrations of blindness or partial sightedness due to diabetic retinopathy in an 18-month period. Of the cases identified, one-quarter were classified as 'failures in diagnosis' (that is, their diabetes had been diagnosed less than 12 months prior to the blindness registration); one-third were due to failure of screening; and just over one-third were classified as treatment failures (either because the condition was not amenable to treatment, or because there was some delay in patients being treated). This sort of audit provides health authorities and trusts with valuable information about the areas where services are failing.

Complications of the feet

121. Health authorities and trusts have a responsibility to provide a comprehensive service that can ensure early detection and treatment of people with foot problems. Only one-third of health authorities surveyed by the Audit Commission provided a district-wide service that offers regular preventative treatment to patients, with speedy referral to specialist foot clinics when problems are detected.

122. Some groups of people with diabetes, such as older people living in residential or nursing homes, may be particularly in need of regular review by podiatrists. Most podiatrists are employed in community settings but few are dedicated to diabetes care, although at sites visited by the Audit Commission, podiatry staff estimated that between 15 and 40 per cent of their workload related to people with diabetes. The problem of variability of access to routine podiatry services is discussed in more detail in the last chapter.

123. Particularly important to good foot care is the early detection and treatment of diabetic foot ulcers. A recent study showed that 5 to 15 per cent of people with diabetic foot ulcers require lower extremity amputation (Ref. 5). At one Audit Commission study site, a review of 25 recent referrals to the specialist foot service found that half were considered by the consultant to have been referred too late for optimum treatment [CASE STUDY 14].

CASE STUDY 14

Clinical audit of foot referrals

At **Kings College Hospital Foot Clinic**, a leading foot service based in London, a retrospective review was carried out of 25 patients. This looked at the mode of referral and time before the patient was seen by staff at the clinic.

The results of the review were as follows:

- Five patients had been referred appropriately by healthcare professionals.

- Twelve patients had been referred late by other health professionals. This included two patients with severe infection who were referred after one week and should have been referred immediately. The average time for referral by healthcare professional was 13 weeks.

- Five patients had referred themselves – these were patients already known to staff at the clinic. One of these patients had waited a week but should have come to the clinic immediately.

- Three further patients were noted to have lesions at their follow-up visit to clinic, but they were unaware of them.

The results of this study were used to develop criteria for appropriate referral, as follows:

- 24 hours if the tissue is inflamed (cellulitis) or dead (necrosis);

- two weeks if ischaemic ulcer unhealed; and

- four weeks if neuropathic ulcer unhealed.

These criteria are being promoted throughout the district to general practices and community staff who make referrals to the hospital foot service.

Key features include:

- highlights inappropriate referrals;

- identifies possible training needs (awareness of referral criteria) for referring staff in the community; and

- highlights deficiencies in foot awareness among patients.

124. Solutions to better foot care include initiatives to educate patients and staff, especially in the community, and the promotion of interdisciplinary guidelines to ensure that referrals are timely and appropriate. Well-funded podiatry services are also needed to ensure regular surveillance of patients and maintenance of good foot health. Some hospitals visited for this study had taken active steps to develop comprehensive foot services for their community [CASE STUDY 15].

CASE STUDY 15

Dealing with complications – foot services

Ipswich General Hospital has a well-established foot clinic that is supported by a multidisciplinary team of medical, nursing, podiatry and orthotic staff. Patients access the service by open referral – usually from the local GP, practice or district nurse. Not all staff are dedicated to the clinic, and some posts are funded by 'soft' monies, like research grants, but the clinic has been able to develop an effective service. As well as the clinical demands of providing a foot service to the diabetic population, the team has developed a series of guidelines and training opportunities for community staff.

One important innovation is patient-held foot records to ensure continuity of care from different professionals. Each time that feet are checked or treatment is given is recorded on a card that the patient keeps.

There is also an emphasis on research and audit. The clinic has carried out a community audit over 12 months showing the kind of foot care that patients receive in a number of settings, including residential homes. There has also been an inpatient audit of bed days for people with foot problems.

Key features include:
- patient-held foot record, to ensure better co-ordination of information across sectors;
- multidisciplinary team with training opportunities for community staff; and
- local audit of foot care in the hospital and in the wider community.

129. The diabetes specialist team has an important role in helping ward staff to improve inpatient care, by providing training, facilitating the development of guidelines, and providing written information for people with diabetes [CASE STUDY 16].

CASE STUDY 16

Inpatient care

People with diabetes who stay as inpatients have particular needs that hospitals should address.

At **Nevill Hall Hospital, Abergavenny**, there is a system of link nurses on each hospital ward. This network provides an opportunity for ward nurses to receive training on diabetes care and be updated on latest developments. These might include changes in insulin delivery for Type 1 patients or techniques for identifying foot problems. There is a structured programme of education for ward nurses devised by the diabetes team. This training is supplemented by a set of guidelines, called the *Diabetes Reference Manual*, which is widely available to ward staff throughout the hospital.

Key features include:

- forum for training and discussion of diabetes issues among ward nurses;

- encouraging professional development for ward nurses; and

- conduit for disseminating changes in diabetes policy and practice throughout the hospital.

The **Royal United Hospital, Bath** has employed a diabetes specialist nurse who is dedicated to inpatient care. She is responsible for educating inpatients with diabetes and staff on all wards. She ensures appropriate diabetes treatment before and after surgery, with interventional procedures where appropriate. In some cases, she can avoid admissions, when patients are seen in acute assessment unit as an emergency. Importantly, this post also acts as a liaison with general practices and/or community diabetes specialist nurses, when patients with diabetes are discharged from hospital care.

Key features include:

- dedicated post to improve co-ordination of diabetes care in hospital;

- avoids unnecessary admission by immediate assessment of emergency cases; and

- liaison with community staff when patients are discharged from hospital.

The diabetes team at **Middlesbrough General Hospital** has produced guidelines for managing people with diabetes in the wards and clinics. These include contact details for all members of the diabetes team and an outline of the processes of care at the diabetes clinic, including the role of the diabetes specialist nurse. Detailed treatment guidelines have been developed in areas ranging from foot care to pregnancy.

The guidance also includes clinic schedules and ends by inviting questions from staff and emphasising that guidelines can only provide pointers to appropriate treatment. The guidance is supported by a system of link nurses and regular training of ward staff. Guidelines were in use on 88 per cent of the wards that were surveyed by the study team at this hospital.

Key features include:

- comprehensive guidance on all aspects of management of patients with diabetes;

- helpful diabetes team contact points for hospital wards; and

- outline of what services the diabetes team offers for patients and staff throughout the hospital.

130. This study has highlighted some key concerns in the management of people with diabetes who are staying in hospital. Many people are diagnosed only once they come into hospital, so it is important that these individuals see a member of the diabetes team and have access to relevant patient information and are followed up after discharge. Links between the diabetes team and hospital wards are often poor and not all places have useful patient information or up-to-date guidelines to help ward staff to provide day-to-day care for their inpatients with diabetes. The principle of supporting self-management by people with diabetes should be encouraged in hospitals as in other settings.

Services for children

131. Mortality rates for people diagnosed with diabetes under the age of 30 are considerably higher than those in the general population (Ref. 51). Type 1 diabetes is the third most common chronic condition in childhood, after asthma and cerebral palsy. The incidence of children with diabetes under 15 is 14.2 per 100,000 per year and there are at least 20,000 children and young adults with diabetes in the UK (Ref. 3). The incidence of children with diabetes appears to be rising, particularly for very young children. One regional study suggested an annual increase for children under 15 of 4 per cent from 1985 to 1996, with an increase of 11 per cent for those under 5 (Ref. 52). The increase in very young children is particularly important, as these children tend to be diagnosed late, to be more severely ill at presentation and to require much longer periods of follow-up in children's clinic. Demands on hospital services are likely to increase markedly in the next few years, given this rising incidence.

132. As in the adult population, good control of blood glucose levels reduces the incidence and delays progression of microvascular complications. Early screening for diabetic complications of kidneys, feet and eyes is now generally recommended from the beginning of puberty. However, the US Diabetes Control and Complications Trial (Ref. 24) showed that achieving tight glycaemic control can be more difficult during puberty. Given the potential for metabolic control to deteriorate during adolescence, good services for young people and close collaboration between paediatric and adult diabetes teams are crucial.

133. The most common cause of death for people with diabetes under the age of 20 is from acute complications of diabetes, namely ketoacidosis and hypoglycaemia. Recent research shows that these death rates have not declined, as might be expected given the experience of other countries and general improvements in care, although absolute numbers of deaths are small (Ref. 51). This points to the need for effective emergency services and ongoing support and education for young people and their families, so that they receive the help that they need to prevent and manage acute episodes.

The incidence of children with diabetes appears to be rising...and demands for hospital services are likely to increase markedly

134. Young people with diabetes should be managed by paediatric specialist diabetes teams and seen in designated children's diabetes clinics. Registers should include comprehensive data on children and their outcomes. In terms of resources, young people and their families require considerable input from a wide range of staff including medical, nursing and psychological support. Recent guidelines (Ref. 53) state that every district must have a consultant paediatrician with a special interest in diabetes and a specialist nurse for children with diabetes (Ref. 54), as well as access to a paediatric dietitian and other specialist staff. The Royal College of Paediatrics and Child Health has also underlined the importance of having designated children's diabetic clinics (Ref. 55).

135. But many places fall short of this ideal. A national survey was carried out which indicated that there were still areas where children were managed in general clinics by paediatricians without specialist interest in diabetes and without the full range of expert support staff, such as specialist nurses, dietitians and psychologists (Ref. 56). A further survey of dietetic provision showed that specialist paediatric dietitians were not available in many places (Ref. 57).

136. At hospitals visited by the Audit Commission, two out of nine did not have an identified paediatrician with a diabetes interest and three of the nine sites had no specialist paediatric diabetes nurse. Two of the nine hospitals had no specialist paediatric dietitian available to the service. In addition, six out of nine had no paediatric psychological or psychiatric input.

137. The diagnosis of diabetes can have a traumatic effect on children and their families and immediate support and counselling is needed. Home visits and 24-hour support from nursing and other staff are particularly important in the care of children, and hospitals need to develop effective outreach links in the community. Paediatric diabetes specialist nurses are particularly important in liaising between the diabetes service and school nurses, health visitors, GPs and practice nurses.

138. In many places, it is routine to admit children to hospital as inpatients when they are diagnosed. The UK St Vincent group on the care of young people with diabetes recommended that 'where the child is admitted to hospital this should be for the shortest time', (Ref. 58) although there is not a clear consensus on best practice. What is clear is that admission and length of stay should be based on the needs of individual patients and their families. Seven out of the nine Audit Commission study sites stated that 80 per cent or more of children are admitted on diagnosis and lengths of stay varied greatly between sites [EXHIBIT 13]. Some sites wanted to shorten hospital stays, but found this difficult because of insufficient nurse resources for home visits, particularly in rural and dispersed areas.

EXHIBIT 13

Admission of children on diagnosis

The usual length of stay in hospital for children just diagnosed with diabetes varied greatly among study sites.

Note: Data presented here for seven out of nine trusts – the other two admitted 15 per cent or less of children on diagnosis.

Source: Audit Commission study sites

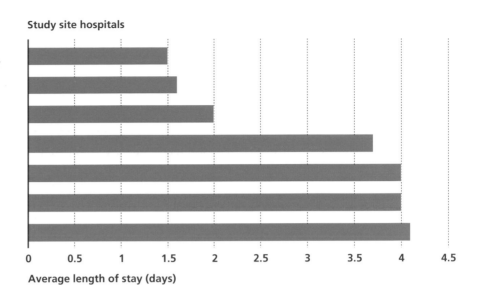

Study site hospitals

Average length of stay (days)

139. Services also need to make special efforts to address the needs of adolescents – a crucial area which poses real challenges. Adolescents are particularly vulnerable, as parental care of diabetes during childhood may not be replaced by equally stringent self-care and many professionals talk about young adults being 'lost to the service' at this time. It is essential that the transfer from paediatric to adult services is smooth and, ideally, tailored to the needs of the individual. There is a variety of approaches in different places and the age of transfer may range from 12 to 18 years, depending on the policy of the trust. Some places organise combined or hand-over clinics, with close links between the paediatric and diabetes teams, to ensure that there is continuity of care for adolescents who are entering the adult diabetes service. Services for adolescents also need particular features – for instance, young women need advance counselling so that they can take steps to prepare themselves for healthy pregnancies.

140. Non-attendance is a particular problem in young adults and the service needs to keep track of its patients and take active steps to maximise attendance. It is dispiriting for staff that sometimes their best efforts do not result in improved attendance rates – although some hospitals have managed to retain regular contact with the great majority of young adults under their care. Approaches which seem to work in some places include reminder telephone calls by the liaison nurse before appointments or changing clinic times to improve access.

...services will increasingly be under pressure to demonstrate [appropriate] clinical governance arrangements...

141. There is now greater recognition of the importance of services for young people with diabetes. A national survey of paediatricians in 1988 showed that almost half of hospitals had no specific clinic facilities for adolescents with diabetes, although by 1994 this proportion had decreased to a third (Ref. 56). The much smaller sample of sites visited by the Audit Commission in 1998/99 suggested that more improvements had taken place since then, with eight out of nine hospitals having some designated clinic or arrangement for young people.

142. There are clear areas for improvement in children's services. A good service can help to generate the lifelong confidence that young people need to manage their condition. The rising incidence among children means that hospital teams are likely to be under increased pressure to support children with diabetes and their families in the future.

Services for pregnant women

143. About four in a thousand pregnant women have Type 1 diabetes. This is not very common and an individual hospital may not see many cases. But in addition, about 1 to 2 per cent of pregnant women develop diabetes during pregnancy ('gestational' diabetes). As well as the complications of pregnancy, up to 60 per cent of women with gestational diabetes will acquire Type 2 diabetes later in life.

144. About one-third of diabetic pregnancies used to end in babies being born dead or dying soon after birth. Despite a dramatic improvement in the last few decades, perinatal mortality is still about four times as high in diabetic pregnancies (56 per 1,000 births) compared with non-diabetic pregnancies (14 per 1,000 births). Other risks to the health of women and babies include increased risk of congenital malformations, ketoacidosis, or diabetic coma, and retinal disease and pregnancy-related complications including pre-eclampsia (Ref. 59).

145. The St Vincent declaration includes a target to achieve pregnancy outcome in the diabetic woman that is similar to that of the non-diabetic woman. Good glycaemic control before and during pregnancy can enable women with diabetes to achieve the same pregnancy outcomes as women without diabetes. There is no consensus about the precise blood glucose levels to aim for in diabetic pregnancy or the best process of maternity care. But the best outcomes seem to be associated with teams that are experienced in managing diabetes in pregnancy and the availability of 24-hour help when problems arise (Ref. 59).

146. The diagnostic criteria for gestational diabetes is an area of some controversy at present (Ref. 60) and health authorities are failing to take the lead. One third of the nine sites visited by the Audit Commission did not have consistent guidelines across the district. Once diagnosed, women with gestational diabetes need considerable education and support. They also need information about reducing the risks of diabetes in later life. Similarly, women with Type 1 diabetes need early counselling to help them to maintain good diabetic control before conception – by trained hospital and general practice staff. But three of the nine sites visited by the Audit Commission did not offer pre-pregnancy counselling for women with diabetes.

147. Pregnant women with Type 1 diabetes are normally cared for by hospital specialists and referred immediately by GPs once pregnancy is diagnosed. Most hospitals offer some form of joint clinic, with input from both maternity and diabetes services. But women who are mainly cared for in hospitals still require support from their GPs and practice nurses in controlling their diabetes and for prescribing, and from midwives. Some women experience shared care between general practice and the hospital – in which case, patient-held records, including details of metabolic control are essential and appear to work well in many places.

148. Babies of women with diabetes may also need special care once they are born. There is variation in practice, with some hospitals routinely admitting all babies born to women with diabetes to the Special Care Baby Unit. The St Vincent Taskforce suggested that 'only a minority with serious neonatal problems will require admission to a neonatal unit' (Ref. 59). Three of the nine hospitals visited by the Audit Commission had a policy of automatic admission, while the others admitted according to need.

149. Services for pregnant women with diabetes showed variation in practice and important gaps, such as the lack of provision of pre-pregnancy counselling at one-third of hospitals visited. Some inconsistencies, such as screening for gestational diabetes, should be reviewed at a national level.

Improving quality

150. This last section considers the 'glue' that binds good diabetes services together. It looks in particular at the information that hospital diabetes services need to review services, initiatives to improve the co-ordination between staff, and ways of enhancing professional development and training within and between disciplines. These are all factors that underpin good care, and services will increasingly be under pressure to demonstrate that they take these activities seriously, as part of clinical governance arrangements in the health service (Ref. 61).

Information and monitoring

151. The importance of information and monitoring was discussed in the last chapter, as part of the responsibilities of those planning services. However, trusts also have responsibilities to monitor:

- processes of care, such as annual review coverage and criteria that affect attendance by patients, such as waiting times;
- intermediate outcomes of care (such as glycaemic control, blood pressure control, as well as measures of patient knowledge);
- use of services (such as hospital admission for ketoacidosis and hypoglycaemia); and

- outcomes of care (including quality-of-life measures and adverse outcomes such as new cases of blindness, amputations and deaths).

152. Many trusts have recognised the importance of good information, and have set in place systems for patient reviews and monitoring routine care. Where this works best, it is linked to a district-wide diabetes register, which also covers patients who receive their review in primary care. Standard forms are used for recording the processes and outcomes of the structured review. This in itself facilitates audit, improves record keeping, and helps continuity of care.

I would like more information about the results of the various blood tests and blood pressure test. I feel somewhat in the dark as to how I am progressing; one is given the impression 'all is well'. How well? Is there more I should be doing? What are the latest developments – could they help me?

153. Reviewing the coverage of annual reviews within the trust and in primary care has enabled the professional staff to identify shortcomings, and address deficiencies. Recording measurements such as blood pressure and blood glucose levels helps to chart long-term control [CASE STUDY 17], and provides an opportunity to open up dialogue with patients about their progress.

154. It is difficult for health authorities and trusts to assess the quality of services without information on clinical and psychological outcomes. But only three of the nine hospitals visited by the Audit Commission could provide data on outcomes such as the number of diabetes-related amputations and admissions for ketoacidosis. Information on new cases of blindness among the diabetic population is particularly poorly recorded. Where registration forms were completed and sent to the Office of National Statistics and then to the Department of Health, the Audit Commission found that there were no arrangements for processing the forms, analysing the data or providing feedback to hospitals. It has been almost ten years since any analysis of this information was available.

155. One specific area of inconsistency across the country is in the monitoring of glycaemic control. It is generally accepted that HbA1c results represent the best single measure of glycaemic control, but not all trusts use this measurement. Where they do, there is no standard assay and reference ranges vary round the country. This hampers comparison by professionals and patients and should be addressed at a national level.

CASE STUDY 17

Information and record keeping

At **Leicester General Hospital**, a system is in place for informing GPs and patients of the results of eye screening. There is an open access eye-screening clinic where patients are sent for retinal photography. Copies of the photographs, report and other test results (HbA1c values, blood pressure values and urine protein results) are sent to the GP *and to the patient*. The report received by the patient and GP includes qualitative assessment and recommendations for future action.

This system of feedback on retinal screening has been evaluated by a postal questionnaire of general practitioners.

The hospital also uses a computer system for its general diabetes consultations, which is designed to be used by all staff. Doctors, nurses, dietitians, podiatrists and receptionists are prompted to carry out certain steps (for example, put eye drops in before examining eyes) and to record the results. Key questions, such as whether the patient has experienced any hypoglycaemic episodes or general problems, are also asked and the answers recorded. The patient is given a printout of the consultation and comments from all staff at the end of the visit and a copy is sent to their GP.

Key features include:

* GP retains comprehensive information on the patient;
* patient is informed of results;
* input from all members of the diabetes team on patient progress; and
* qualitative assessment helps patient to monitor their own health.

Professional links

156. The last chapter considered the steps that could be taken by those planning services to co-ordinate care for people with diabetes across a whole population. This section provides a more detailed examination of some of these problems, focusing mainly on evidence from hospital study sites, and considers some solutions to improve the co-ordination of care. This affects both staff working in different sectors and staff working in different specialties within the hospital.

The doctor/nurse was not aware that I was taken into hospital on the two visits to the diabetic clinic. There was nothing on my notes, which I thought was bad.

157. Poor communication across the primary and secondary care interface has many consequences, including duplication of tests and examinations, or failure to carry out procedures in either setting. A study of a sample of hospital patient notes showed that:

- one in five GP referral letters gave no clear indication of the problem that led to referral;

- one in four letters made no mention of current diabetes control;

- almost half of all letters failed to indicate what interim action had been taken by GPs; and

- over two-thirds of records and letters from hospitals back to GPs failed to note what information had been given to the patient.

158. Communication between primary and secondary care could be improved through joint agreement on the content of referral letters, and patients would benefit from explicit policies on what information should be give to them. Some places have experimented with ways of making information more accessible to patients, as illustrated by Case Study 17. The use of guidelines, electronic patient records and other forms of information-sharing were considered in the last chapter.

I have a feeling of falling between different medics – problems are missed or not acted upon.

159. As well as good communication across sectors, there also needs to be good co-ordination between the diabetes team and other specialties in the hospital, particularly for the treatment of people with complications. These specialties include ophthalmology, vascular surgery, renal medicine, obstetrics and paediatrics. Clinics run jointly by the diabetes team and associated specialists can work very well in providing co-ordinated care to the patient [CASE STUDY 18]. But not all hospitals visited had clear routes of referral for people with urgent complications that require immediate attention.

CASE STUDY 18

Links within the hospital

A key feature of good diabetes care in hospitals is the way in which the diabetes service is linked to other specialties.

At **Kings College Hospital, London**, there is a wide range of joint clinics and special clinics in a range of associated specialties, such as neuropathy, nephropathy (see glossary) and impotence. Most are held weekly. For these joint clinics, specialists (such as neurologists) see patients alongside the diabetologist. In addition, concurrent clinics are held in areas such as ophthalmology on days when diabetes clinics are held. There is a 'one stop shop' for complications, where patients can be seen by renal and eye specialists on the same day.

CASE STUDY 18 (continued)

Special clinics include a leading foot service, which is focused largely on the needs of patients with diabetes. There is good access to vascular surgery and related specialist staff.

Joint working with the maternity service is particularly well developed. Two diabetic consultants, two specialist diabetes nurses, two midwives, two obstetricians and a dietitian staff clinics for pregnant women with diabetes. Women are seen every two weeks to maintain tight control of blood glucose. There is also a pre-pregnancy session for women who are thinking of having babies to stabilise their blood glucose levels, receive folic acid and counselling. Outcomes of pregnancies, such as weight of babies and rate of caesarean sections, are audited and kept under review.

Benefits include:

- range of weekly joint specialist clinics for patients with complications;
- good joint working and speedy referral from diabetes team to specialist services; and
- 'one stop shop' aims to reduce number of hospital visits for patients.

At **Poole Hospital**, there are a range of joint clinics with a focus on patients with complications. By understanding exactly which patients the 'specialist' would want to treat, the diabetologist can ensure that appropriate cases are referred. This also gives the diabetologist greater confidence to manage 'less complicated' cases in their own clinic, knowing that specialist advice is readily available.

One benefit for patients is that clinics for foot care and other complications are all based in the diabetes centre. They can then stay within the diabetes centre for all consultations. This includes specialist eye services, where assessment by the ophthalmologist and laser treatment is also available on site. The centre is an attractive, dedicated premise with comfortable waiting areas and the opportunity to meet other people with diabetes and read information related to their diabetes care.

It also provides an opportunity for specialist staff, such as ophthalmologists, to feel part of the extended diabetes team and to keep up to date with development in diabetes care by being on site (for instance, joining diabetes team staff lunchtime meetings). It also provides good training opportunities for junior doctors and other members of the multidisciplinary diabetes team.

Key features include:

- range of specialist clinics held at the diabetes centre;
- minimises travelling across hospital for patients; and
- gives specialist staff more involvement in diabetes care and provides training opportunities across a range of disciplines.

CASE STUDY 19

Supporting professional development in diabetes care

All staff involved in the care of people with diabetes need training which is up to date and appropriate to their needs.

The **Royal United Hospital, Bath**, supports a primary care team to run diabetes special interest group meetings throughout the district. These are aimed at GPs, practice nurses, district nurses and health visitors and are held in the evenings at different GP surgeries to maximise local attendance.

A popular event run by the diabetes team is a 'hands on' day for GPs and practice nurses. These are focused on particular topics, with emphasis on practical learning. Examples include foot care, with demonstrations of treatments on patients from the foot clinic; a display and demonstration of gadgets used in diabetes care; and eye screening illustrated by patient volunteers, using retinal photography. Staff delivering care in a team – such as a practice nurse and a GP – are encouraged to attend together.

More formal training is offered to staff in general practice and the community. This ranges from a basic three day course, through a classic ENB course (University of the West of England), to a multiprofessional training course over two or three months with a five day training block and a residential weekend (Bath Spa University). The diabetes team provides input to the content of many of these courses. All diabetes courses, special interest meetings and teaching days are fully evaluated, using anonymised return forms. These are used to audit, modify and improve future programmes. Prior PGEA approval is obtained where necessary.

The hospital team runs regular lunchtime meetings for all staff involved in the care of people with diabetes. These include guest speakers, and staff take it in turns to chair the meeting and set the agenda. Practice nurses and district nurses are also encouraged to sit in on hospital diabetes clinics.

Specialist nurses are also involved in a research project to evaluate systematically the impact of structured educational programme for primary care teams. The project involves 18 practices with before and after testing of practice nurses following intensive diabetes training by a specialist nurse.

Key features include:

• mixture of formal and informal training for a wide range of staff in hospital, primary and community care;

• emphasis on practical learning and teambuilding for staff delivering diabetes care; and

• events held at different locations across the trust catchment to maximise participation.

165. Sharing information and skills is especially important for staff who are isolated and for whom diabetes is only a small part of their workload. Residential homes are a particular source of concern, as underlined in a recent report by the BDA (Ref. 65), because of the high overall prevalence of diabetes and the higher than expected rates of complications and use of hospital services for this group. Responsibility for these individuals may not be clear and they may not receive care from staff with expertise in diabetes management. In response to these concerns, some diabetes teams have invested special effort in reaching staff in residential nursing homes [**CASE STUDY 20**] and other environments, such as prisons, where diabetes awareness may not be high.

CASE STUDY 20

Supporting professional development in residential nursing homes

Elderly people living in residential or nursing homes with diabetes are not always well served by existing services.

An initiative at **Middlesbrough General Hospital** has been set up to identify the educational needs for those who look after people with diabetes in nursing homes. This project was initiated by the diabetes liaison nurse, who sent out a questionnaire to managers of nursing homes asking for information about their residents with diabetes and the kinds of support and information about diabetes that was available to staff. Results from the survey highlighted concerns with poor control of diabetes – for instance, 18 per cent of respondents reported recent incidents of hypoglycaemia. A significant proportion did not appear on the district register or local general practice records. The survey also helped to identify areas where staff felt least confident in caring for people with diabetes.

Following this survey, the diabetes team at Middlesborough General Hospital organised a formal study day for staff in residential homes. This was followed up by visits from the liaison nurse to reinforce the training and to check how care was being delivered in practice. Written information for patients and carers was provided for all homes. In addition, guidelines were developed to ensure appropriate treatment and referral.

Key features include:

- awareness of gaps in current provision of care to people with diabetes in residential homes;

- training for staff in residential homes that focused on areas of concern; and

- active links and continuing support between hospital diabetes team and residential homes.

4 ———

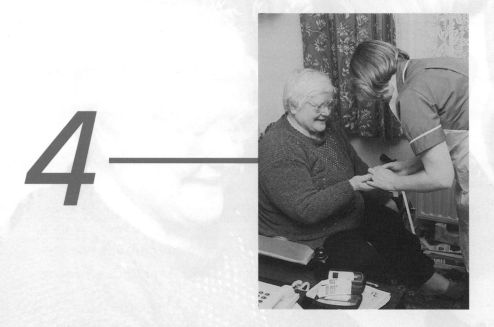

Meeting the Challenges of the 21st Century

Services are under pressure now, and there is considerable variation in staffing levels across the country. Demands will intensify with growing patient numbers and changes in treatments over the coming years. One option is for more routine care to be provided outside hospitals, freeing up specialist diabetes teams to focus on complicated cases and supporting primary and community staff. This has begun to happen in some places and may be the way forward for diabetes care.

Introduction

169. The prospects for people living with diabetes have never been better. Improved control of the condition means that individuals can lead full and active lives, while new developments in insulin and its administration have made everyday management easier. Women with diabetes can, with the right treatment and support, expect to have normal, or near-normal, pregnancies and healthy babies. For all people with diabetes, greater understanding of the condition has underlined the importance of preventing complications and the need for regular assessment. New evidence from the UKPDS has underlined the fact that diabetes is a serious condition and demonstrated that good control can make a real difference in delaying complications. There has also been a shift of focus in recent years, the emphasis now being on how professionals can best support individuals with diabetes in their lifelong task of maintaining their own health and wellbeing.

170. But while there is clear understanding of what needs to be done to maintain good health and support people with diabetes, not all parts of the health service are delivering this. And the task will become more difficult as pressure is placed on over-stretched services to meet growing demands over the next few years. This chapter looks at these growing demands in the light of current provision and considers the changes that may be needed for services to cope.

Pressure on current services

171. What is the evidence on current levels of resources for diabetes services? As discussed in the first chapter, information from published research is scanty – in the words of one commentator, 'for such a chronic and potentially disabling disease with numerous complications, it is surprising that costs have not been more extensively researched' (Ref. 66). What evidence exists is focused on direct costs and tends to measure activity in the hospital sector alone.

172. The main driver for costs in diabetes care, as for most clinical areas, is staffing. The BDA and Royal College of Physicians commissioned a survey of consultant staffing (adjusted for estimates of time spent on diabetes) which was published in 1999 (Ref. 67). This showed great variation in resources, with more than ten-fold difference between the highest and lowest figures [EXHIBIT 14, overleaf]. There are no *evidence-based* standards for optimum staffing levels. However, the BDA has produced recommendations of levels of staffing for various disciplines involved in diabetes care (Ref. 53).[1] These are based on targets set by professional bodies for medical (Ref. 68), nursing (Ref. 69) and other staffing. The national survey of consultant staffing shows that only one district meets current recommended levels set by the profession.

I   Note that recommendations were for catchments of 250,000 and included 28.75 sessions for consultant physicians a week and at least 4.0 WTE specialist nurses, as well as 1.5 dietitians and 2.5 podiatrists for populations of this size.

EXHIBIT 14

Consultant staffing for diabetes care in England and Wales 1999

There was great variation in the levels of consultant staffing.

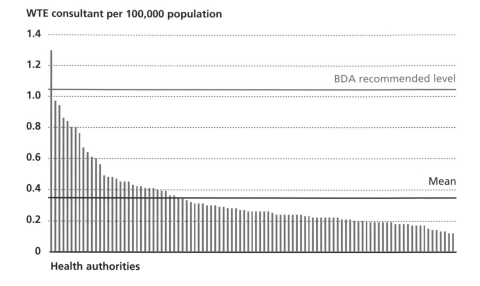

WTE consultant per 100,000 population

BDA recommended level

Mean

Health authorities

Source: BDA staffing survey (1999)

173. There is no equivalent national survey of specialist diabetes nursing, but figures from the Audit Commission study showed that only two out of nine study sites met the recommended specialist nursing standards set by the BDA [**EXHIBIT 15**].[I]

I It is unclear whether BDA standards include community-based diabetes specialist nurses as well – figures from the Audit Commission study sites included all nurses delivering some care in the hospital, whether posts were funded by acute or community trusts. The levels of staffing therefore may be even lower than this Exhibit suggests.

EXHIBIT 15

Levels of specialist nursing at study sites

There was variation between hospitals in the levels of staffing for specialist diabetes nurses.

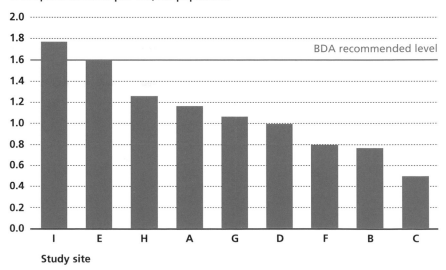

WTE specialist nurse per 100,000 population

BDA recommended level

Study site

Source: Audit Commission study sites

174. A similar picture is seen in a more detailed analysis of consultant and specialist nursing staffing by patients seen at diabetes clinics in hospitals visited by the Audit Commission [**EXHIBIT 16**]. This shows a three- to four-fold variation in medical and nursing staffing at clinics. Different conclusions can be drawn from this and there is no guidance on optimum staffing levels at clinics. However, this small snapshot suggests very different use of specialist staff at different sites, with varying levels of patient contact from hospital to hospital.

175. Other professions involved in diabetes care also show a similar picture of variation in staffing provision. The BDA carried out a survey of dietitians in 1997 and this shows uneven provision across the country (Ref. 40). Eighty-five per cent of dietitians worked in areas where provision was less than the current standard recommended by the BDA, and the median level of dietetic provision overall was less than half of the recommended target.

176. There is also great variation in community podiatry services across the country, with some areas very poorly served (Ref. 70). A recent study by Age Concern found that demand has more than doubled in the last five years, but that podiatry budgets have not kept pace with this increase (Ref. 71). In diabetes care, the Audit Commission survey of general practices revealed that only 27 per cent of GP practices surveyed had access to podiatry services. The Department of Health is currently examining levels of podiatry services as part of its overall workforce planning review.

EXHIBIT 16

Clinic workload and resources

Study of specialist staff and patient workload showed great variation between hospitals.

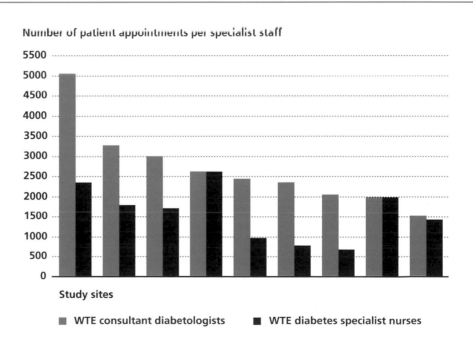

Number of patient appointments per specialist staff

Study sites

■ **WTE consultant diabetologists**   ■ **WTE diabetes specialist nurses**

Source: Audit Commission study sites

Services are finding it hard to cope with current demands...and demands for support, treatments and specialist staff will increase

177. The data supports the view held by many clinicians themselves: services are finding it hard to cope with current demands. But this situation is likely to get worse. The number of people diagnosed with diabetes is likely to increase from 1.4 million to 3 million by the year 2010 (Ref. 8). This represents a more than two-fold increase by the end of this decade. In addition, many people are living with undiagnosed diabetes. More effective case-finding is likely to result in an even larger patient population.

178. Other factors indicate that services will be increasingly under pressure. The recent landmark UKPDS study emphasised the benefits of intensive treatment in reducing adverse effects of diabetes. The findings pointed to the need for tighter targets for blood pressure and blood glucose control than were recommended earlier (Ref. 72). This has resource implications; for instance, more antihypertensive treatments to control blood pressure and more intensive treatment for people with Type 2 diabetes, including greater use of insulin therapy. It is not just treatment costs – people converting to insulin need specialist support (usually from a specialist diabetes nurse) over time to identify the right dose and work with the patient to ensure they are confident about injecting insulin.

179. It is clear that demands for support, treatments and specialist staff will increase. How will services cope in the future within existing resources?

Re-focusing services

180. Earlier parts of this report considered the current balance of care between primary and secondary settings and concluded that there is real diversity in how care is organised in different parts of the country. This is particularly true for people with Type 2 diabetes, who may receive all their care in general practice, all their care in hospital, or some mixture of the two. Different models of care are likely to depend on historic patterns of referral and the preference of individual patients and clinicians.

Where should patients be treated?

181. What is the evidence on the effectiveness and cost-effectiveness of care in different settings? Probably the most reliable source to date is a Cochrane systematic review and meta-analysis (Ref. 73) which compared the management of diabetes in primary and secondary care settings. Only five of the 1,200 studies identified met the inclusion criteria. From the five studies, the authors concluded that *where primary care was well-organised* (with registers, recall and regular review) there was:

- no significant difference in metabolic control (probably best single outcome measure) between patients treated in primary or secondary care;

- no significant difference in diabetes-related hospital admissions for patients treated in primary or secondary care; and

- no significant differences in blood pressure levels between those in primary and secondary care.

182. There is no conclusive evidence about care being 'better' in primary or secondary settings – much will depend on individual clinicians, patients and the models of care that are available in different localities. Patient preferences may be particularly important, given that diabetes is a condition that relies so heavily on self-management by patients. What is important is that care is provided by enthusiastic, well informed professionals, in accordance with patients' wishes and needs, and with good support and back-up if needed.

What is happening in general practice?

183. This study has focused largely on the activities of diabetes teams in hospitals. But many general practices provide excellent routine care for people with diabetes, in a family doctor setting [CASE STUDY 21]. A recent survey of general practices (Ref. 20) showed that 68 per cent described their practice as having a special interest in diabetes. The BDA recently revised its structures and formed a new professional division for primary care staff (Primary Care Diabetes UK), reflecting the growth of diabetes interest and activity in general practice.

CASE STUDY 21

Diabetes care in general practice

There is no one model of good diabetes care in general practice, but many places are providing excellent care for people with diabetes. Examples such as the one below may not be so easy to replicate in areas with different population catchments, resources and staffing.

St Leonards Medical Practice is a well-established five-doctor practice in central Exeter with a registered population of 6,200 patients, including 152 people with diabetes. The practice is run on the basis of personal lists and the care of people with diabetes is shared among the partners. The population served by the practice is very stable, with the median length of registration being 11 years.

There is no diabetes clinic as such, but patients are seen every four months in a shared appointment between their own GP and the practice nurse. The centre has three practice nurses, one of whom has completed a specialist diabetes course. Each nurse sees an equal number of patients with diabetes and considers diabetes and its management to be one of her core functions. Recall appointments are generated by the computer and patients are reminded after four months if they have not attended. Overall, non-attendance rates are low. Housebound patients are visited by their GP and the community nurse at home.

Continued overleaf

CASE STUDY 21 (continued)

At each appointment or visit, the patient is weighed, their blood pressure and a random blood glucose is taken. An assessment of glycaemic control is also taken at each visit and discussed with the patient as well as general education about their health. Over the year, each person with diabetes will receive full screening for possible complications involving the eyes, kidneys, feet and blood vessels. The 'annual' review therefore takes place across the year but is systematically recorded.

The practice places great emphasis on the importance of good quality information, with a comprehensive database of all its patients. This includes a summary of their medical history, including physical, psychological and social data. The practice is also committed to reviewing its services for patients with diabetes and an audit is run every six months with standards for each criteria that are set and agreed by the partners. They have compared individual doctor's performance in diabetes care using personal list comparisons of glycaemic control, which are used to prompt discussion and informal peer review. The practice has also been able to document rises in prevalence, with the numbers of patients with diabetes having doubled in the last ten years.

Key features include:

- patients are seen by their personal doctor, who has knowledge of their family history and health;

- systematic review provided throughout the year through regular appointments that are convenient to patient; and

- emphasis on information and audit – data on diabetes outcomes by doctor and peer review helps to identify areas for improvement.

184. As well as providing first-line care for people with diabetes, many practices are now offering more extensive diabetes care. This may be the result of a local initiative by an individual practice, or part of a systematic plan by PCGs, LHGs or health authorities [CASE STUDY 22].

Promoting community-based diabetes care

Initiatives in different parts of the country show that more services for people with diabetes could be provided outside the hospital setting, given the right support.

Ladywood Primary Care Group, in Birmingham, is piloting a project aiming to provide seamless, comprehensive care for the diabetes population that it covers. Patients with uncomplicated diabetes will be seen in general practice mini-clinics, run by a GP and the practice nurse. Shared care will be provided for patients with more complicated diabetes at a consultant-led community clinic. It is envisaged that only a small proportion of patients will continue to attend the acute trust for diabetes care.GPs and practice nurses who wish to take on contracts to run mini-clinics must complete the University of Warwick Primary Care Unit certificate in primary diabetes care. A GP facilitator is leading the project implementation.

The scheme is supported by the health authority which is funding an information system that will be used:

- to collect information on all patients;
- to generate and feed back activity and outcome data; and
- as a call/recall system for eye screening and routine reviews.

Key features include:

- explicit responsibilities for primary and secondary care professionals;

- confidence in high quality general practice care as a result of training;
- improved information about the diabetes population;
- better communication between professionals; and
- consistency of standards of care for patients.

Frome general practice in Somerset has developed a comprehensive diabetes service. This is a large dynamic practice, with a patient list of 26,500 of which about five hundred have diabetes. Staff at the practice were concerned about the services from local hospitals including waiting times, the distance patients had to travel, the duplication of tests and a lack of clear division of responsibilities between GP and hospital service. From November 1997, Frome practice developed an enhanced GP service for diabetes, buying in outside help as needed.

A weekly clinic is held for *all* their patients with diabetes, including those who are insulin-dependent and poorly controlled. The only exclusions are children and pregnant women. The practice contracts for the following outside help:

- a consultant session twice a month (the consultant sitting in with GPs and offering advice on case conferences, rather than actually seeing patients);

- one diabetes specialist nurse for a session every week – offering advice and support to practice nurses and seeing some patients (for instance, those Type 2 patients who are switching to insulin);
- one podiatrist for two sessions a month; and
- one dietitian for two sessions a month.

In the practice, six GPs are involved (with two on a rota for each clinic), a practice nurse and a clinic receptionist. The clinic receptionist offers a key call/recall service. At each clinic, the patient is given their next appointment and an appointment for blood tests three weeks before. The local hospital pathology laboratory downloads results directly to the practice by computer, which provides information about the patients' blood glucose levels before they are seen by the nurse and doctor. GPs refer directly to the eye clinic and the vascular service at the hospital.

Key features include:

- convenience for patients in having a comprehensive local service;
- family doctors see diabetes care in context of patient's 'whole care';
- specialist outreach service by hospital diabetes team; and
- duplication of tests and checks by general practice and hospital is minimised.

What will happen in the future?

185. The variation in the proportion of patients cared for in hospital centres suggests that, with the right support, there is the potential for shifting the balance of care to the community. Such a shift should reflect the particular strengths of primary and secondary care settings, [BOX N] and should always be considered in the context of local circumstances.

BOX N

Strengths of primary and secondary care settings

Strengths of hospital diabetes teams include:

- providing specialist care for people with complications or special groups of patients (such as children and pregnant women);

- providing second-line treatment for patients with poor diabetes control;

- providing expert support and training for all staff in the catchment who care for people with diabetes (including practice nurses, GPs, health visitors, community podiatrists and dietitians);

- providing specialist patient education for a critical mass of patients, including those with special needs (such as ethnic minority groups), and providing input from a range of disciplines; and

- providing a focus for diabetes care in the hospital, including training for hospital staff, guidelines for inpatient care and links with key specialist teams including ophthalmology, vascular surgery and nephrology.

Strengths of primary care teams include:

- continuity of care for the patient;

- knowledge of the patient 'from cradle to grave', the patient's family, and co-morbidities which may affect the course of their diabetes;

- expertise in managing chronic condition;

- services often nearer to home for the patient; and

- may be preferred by patients for routine care. (Ref. 74)

Source: Audit Commission

...more routine care will need to be provided by primary care teams in the future

186. Increased demand makes it likely that more routine care for people with diabetes will need to be provided by primary care teams in the future. Any shift in the balance of care will take time, and changes may be more rapid in some parts of the country than others. In some places, such as Bradford (see Case Study 1, p27) or Birmingham (see Case Study 22), there has been a concerted strategy to provide enhanced diabetes services in the primary care setting. But in many places, local circumstances mean that hospital services will need to continue to provide basic support to many people with diabetes. For instance, results from the Audit Commission survey showed that more than half of patients with diabetes on general practice lists in an area where primary care was less well developed usually see their hospital doctor for routine care. Patterns of care in places like these cannot be altered overnight.

187. But some sites visited for this study have shown that specialist diabetes teams can shift their focus to concentrate on supporting staff in primary and community settings [CASE STUDY 23]. Much of this depends on enthusiastic and committed individuals who have provided a catalyst for change locally.

CASE STUDY 23

Hospitals supporting diabetes care in the community

Hospital diabetes teams in the future will need to play a major role in supporting diabetes care in the community.

The Diabetes Resource Centre at **North Tyneside** has developed a 'community-focused' secondary care service. Funding is mixed, coming partly from health authority, trust (combined acute and community) and voluntary monies. The diabetes team sees its main role as training, supporting and enabling primary care staff to deliver routine care and providing specialist services for people with complications.

There is a strong focus on *patient education*. A psychologist has led a behaviour change project, working with diabetes staff to develop counselling and education skills. The psychologist provides different levels of training in counselling – basic training for most staff (including podiatrists and GPs) and an advanced course for diabetes advisers such as dietitians, specialist nurses and diabetologists. Once staff at the Centre become confident in new skills or new programmes, these are routinely 'rolled out' to primary care.

The Centre has produced a series of *protocols* (for example, screening for renal problems), guidelines (for example, when to start putting patients on insulin) and some supported guidelines (for example, how to set up a GP clinic for diabetes) that aim to improve the consistency of care.

Continued overleaf

Appendix 3

Initiatives to set standards in diabetes care

British Diabetic Association (BDA) and UKDIABS project

The BDA is a well-established patient and professional organisation which campaigns for improvements in care, raises awareness of diabetes, and is a major sponsor of clinical research. The BDA has been a major force in pushing for improved standards of care; for instance, issuing a leaflet to patients on 'what to expect' from health services. It is estimated that membership represents about 10 per cent of the total population of people with diabetes. On the professional side, a new division has recently been formed for primary care staff.

The BDA initiated the UKDIABS project in 1996 with the aim of providing better information on diabetes to districts and clinicians. The project collects data from districts in a standardised form. It now collects information from over one-third of all districts, although some have found it difficult to obtain the relevant data from existing systems.

The BDA has also funded the DIABQoL+ project from 1998 with the aim of developing a range of short reliable instruments to measure psychological outcomes and processes of diabetes care which would be valid for use in routine clinical practice and for audit purposes. Instruments include measures of patient satisfaction with the service provided (DCSQ) and measures of the impact of diabetes on quality of life (ADDQoL). Versions of these measures are already in widespread use while efforts to shorten them continue.

St Vincent Declaration (1989)

The St Vincent Declaration (1989) was an agreement of all European countries, under the auspices of the World Health Organisation and International Diabetes Federation, to improve care for people with diabetes. The importance of psychological well-being, self-care, patient education and community support was emphasised. There were also goals to develop comprehensive programmes for detection and control of diabetes and its complications. In addition, the declaration stated the need for centres of excellence in diabetes care, education and research.

Specific targets were set for the prevention of complications, including:

- reducing new blindness due to diabetes by one-third or more;
- reducing the numbers of people entering end-stage diabetic renal failure by at least one-third;
- reducing the rate of limb amputations for diabetic gangrene by half;
- reducing morbidity and mortality from coronary heart disease in the diabetic population; and
- achieving pregnancy outcome in women with diabetes that approximates to that of non-diabetic women.

The Department of Health/BDA St Vincent Joint Task Force for Diabetes reported in 1995 on progress in these areas and made recommendations about good clinical and management practice in 11 key areas.

Clinical Standards Advisory Group (1994)

Produced an influential report assessing diabetes care in 1994, focused mainly on hospitals. The Clinical Standards Advisory Group was disbanded in 1998, in the light of new Government initiatives to monitor quality in healthcare.

Health Service Guidelines. Key Features of a Good Diabetes Service (1997-1998). HSG(97)45 and Welsh Office WHC(98)35

In 1997 (England) and 1998 (Wales), guidance was issued to health authorities and GP fundholders. This set out general principles of good practice, such as the need for a seamless service working across boundaries.

Joint Royal Colleges Assessment Framework for diabetes (2001)

The BDA, together with the Royal College of Nursing, Royal College of General Practitioners and Royal College of Physicians is developing a comprehensive performance framework for diabetes care. The framework can be used as a whole or in part, depending on local requirements. It is intended to be used for self-assessment and external peer review and is expected to be finalised in 2001.

National Service Framework (NSF) for Diabetes (2001)

A framework to set standards for diabetes care will be published in the year 2001. Performance will be monitored by the Commission for Health Improvement, the National Performance Assessment Framework and the National Survey of Patients.

Hyperglycaemia	High blood glucose level, when the individual has too little insulin.
Hyperglycaemic episodes ('Hyper')	Crisis when patient's blood glucose levels are too high, as a result of untreated or poorly controlled diabetes, missed insulin injections or due to infection. May result in serious diabetic coma. *See* ketoacidosis.
Hypoglycaemia	Low blood glucose level, when the individual has too much insulin.
Hypoglycaemic episodes ('Hypo')	Crisis when patients blood glucose levels drop too low, as a result of excessive doses of insulin, inadequate food or sudden exercise. May lead to loss of consciousness and convulsions.
Incidence	The number of new cases of a disease occurring per unit population per year. (Difficult to ascertain for Type 2 diabetes due to the sometimes long delays between onset and diagnosis.)
Insulin	A pancreatic hormone which controls levels of blood glucose.
Insulin-dependent diabetes mellitus (IDDM)	Type of diabetes that must be treated with insulin; now known as Type 1 diabetes. NB: It is easier to use the terms Type 1 and Type 2 diabetes, as some people with Type 2 diabetes may become dependent on insulin as the condition progresses.
Ischaemia	Insufficient blood supply to part of the body – usually because of blood vessel disease.
Ketoacidosis	Severe case of hyperglycaemia resulting from lack of insulin which, in turn, results in body fat being used to produce energy, forming ketones in the urine, vomiting, drowsiness, heavy laboured breathing and a smell of acetone on the breath. *See* hyperglycaemia.
LDSAG	Local Diabetes Services Advisory Group – a group with professional and user representatives usually reporting to the health authority.
Local health groups – LHGs	Welsh equivalent of a PCG (see primary care groups).
Macrovascular complications	Where the large arteries to the heart, brain, legs and feet become narrow or blocked.
Microvascular complications	Damage to the small blood vessels of parts of the body like eyes, nerves, feet.
Morbidity	The state of being diseased.
National Service Framework (NSF)	Each NSF is developed using a multidisciplinary external reference group, with the aim of ensuring consistency of services, reducing variation in standards of care, setting national standards and defining models of care for diabetes services. Diabetes will be the subject of the next National Service Framework (NSF) for England, to be published in spring 2001.
Nephropathy	Kidney damage or renal problems; initially this causes the kidney to 'leak' so that albumin appears in the urine. Later it may affect kidney function and in severe cases lead to kidney failure.
Nephrologist	Doctor specialising in diseases of the kidney.
Neurologist	Doctor specialising in diseases of the nervous system.
Neuropathy	Damage affecting the nerves.

Non-insulin-dependent diabetes mellitus (NIDDM)	Type of diabetes that usually occurs in older people (usual onset >40 years, but younger in some ethnic groups), particularly if overweight. These people do not always need insulin treatment and can often be controlled successfully with diet alone or diet and drugs. The term more commonly used now is Type 2 diabetes.
Ophthalmologist	Medical specialist in disease and defects of the eye.
Optician/optometrist	Non-medical specialists in eye care.
Orthopaedic surgeons	Surgeon specialising in abnormalities, diseases and injuries of locomotor system.
Orthotist	Technical specialist who assesses footwear needs. Usually works in conjunction with foot clinic.
Patterns of care	The configuration of where patients are treated (usually primary or secondary care settings).
Perinatal	Relating to the period around birth.
PGEA	Postgraduate education allowance – money claimed by GPs for events and courses which are considered to be part of their professional development.
Podiatry/podiatrist	Synonymous with chiropody – for most purposes. Becoming the preferred term among professionals. *See* chiropody.
Prevalence	Number of cases of a disease per unit population at any given time.
Primary care	Usually used to describe first-line services, provided by primary care teams (general practitioners and practice nurses) as well as district nurses, health visitors and a range of community-based staff
Primary care groups – PCGs	Primary care groups were formed on 1 April 1999. They bring together all local general practices and community nurses under a board with social services, health authority and lay representation to promote the health of the local population; commission hospital and community-based health services; and develop primary healthcare.
Psychologist	Non-medical professional, with post graduate training and qualification – specialising in the mind and mental processes.
Random blood glucose	Diabetes can be diagnosed by a random blood glucose level (as opposed to a fasting blood glucose).
Renal physicians	*See* nephrologist.
Retinal screening	Process of surveillance to detect early signs of diabetic retinopathy.
Retinopathy	Problems affecting the retina, the light-sensitive part at the back of the eye which transmits visual images to the brain.
Screening	The carrying out of tests to identify diseases or abnormalities in people before symptoms appear. May be population-based or targeted.

Secondary care	Term usually used to define specialist care, often provided in hospitals. Highly specialised hospital services are known as 'tertiary care'.
Secondary prevention	Term usually used to describe activities to limit the impact of a disease – for example, screen for complications (primary refers to prevention of the disease per se).
Serum cholesterol	Lipid found in blood – high levels are a risk factor for coronary heart disease, and are also indicative of poorly controlled diabetes.
Shared care	A formal arrangement by which the division of responsibility between primary care and secondary care is set down. The definition is not clear and shared care can be interpreted in many different ways.
St Vincent Declaration	International task force which sets standards for diabetes care.
Surveillance	More general term than screening, to describe oversight of a population in order to detect disease and prevent further problems.
Type 1 diabetes	Another name for insulin-dependent diabetes.
Type 2 diabetes	Another name for non-insulin-dependent diabetes.
UKDIABS	BDA/Department of Health-sponsored research project to develop a data system for monitoring diabetes care. Due to be complete in 2002.
UKPDS – United Kingdom Prospective Diabetes Study	A recently published longitudinal study which demonstrated the benefits of tight blood glucose and blood pressure control in preventing complications in Type 2 diabetes.
Visual acuity	Test of vision – usually by means of reading a Sneller chart of characters of diminished size.

Source: Audit Commission, adapted from Mackinnon M, Providing Diabetes Care in General Practice, Class Press, 1998.

References

1. UK Prospective Diabetes Study Group, 'Overview of Six Years' Therapy of Type 2 Diabetes: – A Progressive Disease (UKPDS 16)', *Diabetes*, Vol. 44, 1995, pp1249-58.

2. Pickup J, Williams G, *Textbook of Diabetes*, 2nd edn., Blackwell Science, 1997.

3. British Diabetic Association, *Diabetes in the UK 1996*, British Diabetic Association, 1995.

4. Viberti G C et al, 'Report on Renal Disease in Diabetes', *Diabetic Medicine*, Vol. 13, suppl. 4, 1996, ppS6-S12.

5. Effective Health Care Bulletin, 'Complications of Diabetes', *University of York NHS Centre for Reviews and Dissemination*, Effective Health Care Bulletin, Vol. 5, No. 4, pp1-12.

6. Yudkin J S et al, 'Prevention and Management of Cardiovascular Disease in Patients with Diabetes: An Evidence Base', *Diabetic Medicine*, Vol. 13, suppl. 4, 1996, ppS101-S121.

7. Fox C and Mackinnon M, 'Vital Diabetes', *Class Health*, 1999.

8. Amos A F, McCarty D J, Zimmet P, 'The Rising Global Burden of Diabetes and Its Complications; Estimates and Projections to the Year 2010', *Diabetic Medicine*, Vol. 14, suppl. 5, 1997, pps1-85.

9. World Health Organisation, *Definition, Diagnosis and Classification of Diabetes Mellitus and Its Complications: Report of A World Health Organisation Collaboration*, WHO, 1999.

10. Simmons D et al, 'The Coventry Diabetes Study: Prevalence of Diabetes and Impaired Glucose Tolerance in Europids and Asians', *Quarterly Journal of Medicine*, Vol. 81, 1991, pp1021-30.

11. Laing W and Williams R, *Diabetes: A Model for Health Care Management*, Office of Health Economics, 1989.

12. National Casemix Office, 1995/96 *National Statistics*, Stationery Office, 1997.

13. Alexander W D, 'Diabetes Care in A UK Health Region: Activity, Facilities and Costs', *Diabetic Medicine*, Vol. 5, no. 6, 1988, pp577-81.

14. Currie C J et al, 'Patterns of In and Out Patient Activity for Diabetes: A District Survey', *Diabetic Medicine*, Vol. 13, No. 3, 1996, pp273-80.

15. Currie C J et al, 'NHS Acute Sector Expenditure for Diabetes: The Present, the Future and Excess In-patient Cost of Care', *Diabetic Medicine*, Vol. 14, No. 8, 1997, pp686-92.

16. UK Prospective Diabetes Study Group, 'Intensive Blood Glucose Control with Sulphonylureas or Insulin Compared with Conventional Treatment and Risk of Complications in Patients with Type 2 Diabetes (UKPDS 33)', *The Lancet*, Vol. 352, 1998, pp837-53.

17.   UK Prospective Diabetes Study Group, 'Quality of Life in Type 2 Diabetic Patients is Affected by Complications Not By Intensive Policies to Improve Blood Glucose or Blood Pressure Control (UKPDS 37)', *Diabetes Care*, Vol. 22, No. 7, 1999, pp1125-36.

18.   Department of Health, *The New NHS: Modern, Dependable*, Cm 3807, Stationery Office, 1997.

19.   Wells S, Bennet I, Holloway G, Harlow V, 'Area-wide Diabetes Care: The Manchester Experience with Primary Healthcare Teams 1991-1997', *Diabetic Medicine*, Vol. 15, suppl. 3, 1998, ppS49-53.

20.   Pierce M, Agarwal G and Ridout D, 'The State of Two Nations: Diabetes Care in General Practice in England and Wales', *British Journal of General Practice*, In Press [2000].

21.   Audit Commission, *First Assessment: A Review of District Nursing Services in England and Wales*, Audit Commission, 1999.

22.   Griffin S, 'Diabetes Care in General Practice: Meta-analysis of Randomised Control Trials', *British Medical Journal*, Vol. 317, 1997, pp390-6.

23.   UK Prospective Diabetes Study Group, 'Cost Effectiveness Analysis of Improved Blood Pressure Control in Hypertensive Patients with Type 2 Diabetes (UKPDS 40)', *British Medical Journal*, Vol. 317, 1998, pp720-26.

24.   Diabetes Control and Complications Trial (DCCT) Research Group. 'The Effect of Intensive Treatment of Diabetes on the Development and Progression of Longterm Complications in Insulin-Dependent Diabetes Mellitus', *New England Journal of Medicine*, Vol. 329, 1993, pp977-86.

25.   UK Prospective Diabetes Study Group, 'Tight Blood Pressure Control and Risk of Macrovascular and Microvascular Complications in Type 2 Diabetes (UKPDS 38)', *British Medical Journal*, Vol. 317, 1998, pp703-13.

26.   Alexander W et al, 'The Report of the Clinical Care Group', *Diabetic Medicine*, Vol. 13, suppl. 4, 1996, ppS90-100.

27.   Department of Health, *Key Features of A Good Diabetes Service*, Health Service Guidance HSG(97)45, 1997.

28.   Welsh Office, *Key Features of A Good Diabetes Service*, Welsh Health Circular WHC(98)35, 1998.

29.   Prescott-Clarke P and Primatesta P, *Health Survey for England 1997*, Stationery Office, 1999.

30.   Home P, Coles J, Goldacre M, Mason A, Wilkinson E (eds), *Health Outcome Indicators: Diabetes Report of a working group to the Department of Health*, National Centre for Health Outcomes Development, 1999.

31. Krans H M J et al (eds), *Diabetes Care and Research in Europe: The St Vincent Declaration Action Programme*, World Health Organisation (2nd edition), 1995.

32. Speight J, Barendse S, Bradley C, 'The DIABQoL+ Programme', *Proceedings of the British Psychological Society*, Vol. 7, suppl 1, 1999, p35.

33. Audit Commission, *PCG Agenda: Early Progress of Primary Care Groups in the New NHS*, Audit Commission, 2000. Full report available electronically.

34. D'Costa D F, Samanta A and Burden A C, 'Epidemiology of Diabetes in UK Asians: A Review', *Practical Diabetes*, Vol. 8, No. 2, 1991, pp64-6.

35. Hawthorne K, 'Asian Diabetics Attending a British Hospital Clinic: A Pilot Study to Evaluate their Care', *British Journal of General Practice*, vol. 40, 1990, pp243-7.

36. Wilson E, Wardle EV, Chandel P, Walford S , 'Diabetes Education: An Asian Perspective', *Diabetic Medicine*, Vol. 10, No. 2, 1993, pp177-80.

37. Greenhalgh T, Helman C, Chowdhury A M, 'Health Beliefs and Folk Models of Diabetes in British Bangladeshis: A Qualitative Study', *British Medical Journal*, Vol. 316, 1998, pp978-83.

38. Lindsey J, Jagger C, Hibbert MJ et al, 'Knowledge, Uptake and Availability of Health and Social Services among Asian Gujerati and White Elderly Persons', *Ethnicity and Health*, vol. 2, pp59-69.

39. British Diabetic Association, *What To Expect*, BDA, 1997. Note: available free from the BDA Distribution Unit (telephone: 0800 585088).

40. Nelson M et al, *Survey of Dietetic Provision for Patients with Diabetes 1997*, data on file at the British Diabetic Association and paper submitted for publication.

41. Long-term Medical Conditions Alliance, *Patients Influencing Purchasers*, NHS Confederation, 1997.

42. Department of Health, *Saving Lives: Our Healthier Nation*, Cm 4386, Stationery Office, 1999.

43. Griffin S, Kinmonth A L, Skinner C, Kelly J, *Educational and Psychosocial Interventions for Adults with Diabetes*, British Diabetic Association, 1998.

44. Barendse S et al, 'Closing the Audit Loop with the Diabetes Clinic Satisfaction Questionnaire (DCSQ): Reducing Sources of Dissatisfaction and Increasing Clinician Sensitivity to Patients' Views', *Diabetic Medicine*, Vol.16, suppl.1, 1999, p15.

45. Griffin S J, 'Lost to Follow Up: The Problem of Defaulters from Diabetes Clinics', *Diabetic Medicine*, Vol. 15, suppl. 3, 1998, ppS14-S24.

46. Lustman P J et al, 'Depression in Adults with Diabetes', *Diabetes Care*, Vol. 15, 1992, pp1631-9.

47. Bradley C and Gamsu D S, 'Guidelines for Encouraging Psychological Well-being: Report of a Working Group of the World Health Organisation and St Vincent Declaration Action Programme for Diabetes', *Diabetic Medicine*, Vol. 11, 1994, pp510-16.

48. See, for example, Petterson et al, 'Well-being and Treatment Satisfaction in Older People with Diabetes', *Diabetes Care*, Vol. 21, 1998, pp930-35.

49. Department of Health Clincal Standards Advisory Group, *Standards of Clinical Care for People with Diabetes*, HMSO, 1994.

50. Early Treatment Diabetic Retinopathy Study Research Group, 'Early Photocoagulation for Diabetic Retinopathy: ETDRS report number 9', *Ophthalmology*, Vol. 98, 1991, pp766-85.

51. Laing SP et al, 'The British Diabetic Association Cohort Study, II: Cause-Specific Mortality in Patients with Insulin-Treated Diabetes Mellitus', *Diabetic Medicine*, Vol.16, 1999, pp1-7.

52. Gardner S G et al, 'Rising Incidence of Insulin-Dependent Diabetes in Children Aged under Five Years in the Oxford Region: Time Trend Analysis', *British Medical Journal*, Vol. 315, 1997, pp713-17.

53. British Diabetic Association, *Recommendations for the Structure of Specialist Diabetes Care Services*, BDA, 1999.

54. For more detailed description, see Royal College of Nursing of the UK, *The Role and Qualifications of the Nurse Specialising in Paediatric Diabetes*, Royal College of Nursing, 1998.

55. British Paediatric Association, 'The Organisation of Services for Children with Diabetes in the UK (Report of the BPA Working Party)' *Diabetic Medicine*, Vol. 7, 1990, pp457-64.

56. Haines L C, Swift P G F, 'Report of the 1994 BPA/BDA Survey of Services for Children with Diabetes: Changing Patterns of Care', *Diabetic Medicine*, Vol. 14, 1997, pp693-7.

57. Waldron S, Swift PG F, 'A Survey of the Dietary Management of Children's Diabetes', *Diabetic Medicine*, Vol. 14, 1997, pp698-702.

58. Betts P et al, 'The Care of Young People with Diabetes (St Vincent and Improving Diabetes Care Specialist UK Workgroup Reports)', *Diabetic Medicine*, Vol. 13, suppl. 4, 1996, ppS54-9.

59. Jardine Brown C et al, 'Report of the Pregnancy and Neonatal Care Group (St Vincent and Improving Diabetes Care Specialist UK Workgroup Reports)', *Diabetic Medicine*, vol. 13, suppl. 4, 1996, ppS43-53.

60. Rey E, 'Screening for Gestational Diabetes Mellitus', *British Medical Journal*, Vol. 319, 1999, pp798-9.

61. Department of Health, *Clinical Governance in the NHS*, HSC 1999/65, Department of Health, 1999.

62. Speight J, Barendse S and Bradley C, 'The ADKnowl: Identifying and Understanding Diabetes-specific Knowledge Deficits in Patients and Clinicians', *Diabetic Medicine*, Vol. 16, suppl. 1, p.52.

63. British Dietetic Association, *The Extended Role of the Dietitian*, 1999.

64. Department of Health, *Continuing Professional Development, Quality in the New NHS*, HSC 1999/154, 1999.

65. British Diabetic Association, *Guidelines of Practice for Residents with Diabetes in Care Homes*, BDA, 1999.

66. Leese B, 'The Costs of Diabetes and its Complications', *Soc Sci Med*, Vol. 35, No. 10, pp1303–10.

67. British Diabetic Association, '1999 Manpower Survey', *Diabetes Update*, BDA, Autumn 1999, pp12-15.

68. Royal College of Physicians, *Consultant Physicians: Working for Patients*, Royal College of Physicians,1999.

69. Royal College of Nursing, *The Role of the Diabetes Specialist Nurse*, Royal College of Nursing of the United Kingdom, 1991.

70. Harvey I, Frankel S, Marks R, Shalom D, Morgan M, 'Foot Morbidity and Exposure to Chiropody: Population Based Study', *British Medical Journal*, Vol. 315,1997, pp1054-5.

71. Age Concern, *On Your Feet! – Older People and NHS Chiropody Services*, Age Concern, 1997.

72. Mogensen C E, 'Combined High Blood Pressure and Glucose in Type 2 Diabetes: Double Jeopardy', *British Medical Journal*, Vol. 317, pp693-4.

73. Griffin S and Kinmonth A L, 'Diabetes Care: The Effectiveness of Systems for Routine Surveillance for People with Diabetes', Vol. 4, 1997, pp1-13.

74. For example, evidence showing patient preference for care in general practice setting from: Diabetes Integrated Care Evaluation Team, 'Integrated Care for Diabetes: Clinical, Psychosocial and Economic Evaluation', *British Medical Journal*, Vol. 308, 1994, pp1208-12.

Index References are to paragraph numbers, Boxes, Case Studies and Appendices

Parkin, F. (1979) *Marxist Class Theory: A Bourgeois Critique*. London: Tavistock.

Perez, C. (1985) 'Micro-electronics, long-waves and world structural systems: new perspectives for developing countries', *World Development*, 13 (3).

Pevsner, N. (1960) *Pioneers of Modern Design: From William Morris to Walter Gropius*. Harmondsworth: Penguin.

Pfeil, F. (1995) *White Guys: Studies in Postmodern Domination and Difference*. London: Verso.

Phillips, D.C. (1987) *Philosophy, Science and Social Enquiry: Contemporary Methodological Controversies in Social Science and Related Applied Fields of Research*. Oxford: Pergamon Press.

Piore, M.J. and Sabel, C.F. (1984) *The Second Industrial Divide: Possibilities for Prosperity*. New York: Basic Books.

Plant, S. (1992) *Most Radical Gesture*. London: Routledge.

Pollert, A. (ed.) (1991) *Farewell to Flexibility?* Oxford: Blackwell.

Portwood, D. (1985) 'Careers and redundancy', *The Sociological Review*, 33 (3): 449–68.

Proctor, I. and Padfield, M. (1999) 'Work orientations and women's work: a critique of Hakim's theory of the heterogeneity of women', *Gender, Work and Organization*, 4 (3): 152–62.

Ransome, P.E. (1992) *Antonio Gramsci: A New Introduction*. Hemel Hempstead: Harvester Wheatsheaf.

Ransome, P.E. (1995) *Job Security and Social Stability: The Impact of Mass Unemployment on Expectations of Work*. Aldershot: Ashgate.

Ransome, P.E. (1996) *The Work Paradigm: A Theoretical Investigation of Concepts of Work*. Aldershot: Ashgate.

Ransome, P.E. (1999) *Sociology and the Future of Work: Contemporary Discourses and Debates*. Aldershot: Ashgate.

Richards, J. 'National identity in British wartime films', in: P.M. Taylor (ed.). pp. 42–61.

Richards, T. (1991) *The Commodity Culture of Victorian England: Advertising and Spectacle, 1851–1914*. London: Verso.

Ritzer, G. (1996) *The McDonaldization of Society: An Investigation into the Changing Character of Contemporary Social Life*. London: Pine Forge Press.

Ritzer, G. (2001) *Explorations in the Sociology of Consumption: Fast Food, Credit Cards and Casinos*. London: Sage.

Roberts, J. (ed.) (1994) *Art Has No History: The Making and Unmaking of Modern Art*. London: Verso.

Rojek, C. (1995) *Decentring Leisure: Rethinking Leisure Theory*. London: Sage.

Rojek, C. (2000) *Leisure and Culture*. Basingstoke: Macmillan.

Rojek, C. and Turner, C. (ed.) (1993) *Forget Baudrillard?*. London: Routledge.

Rowbotham, S. (1998) 'Weapons of the weak; homeworkers' networking in Europe', *European Journal of Women's Studies*, 5: 453–63.

Rowe, D. (1999) *Sport, Culture and the Media: The Unruly Trinity.* Buckingham: Open University Press.

Rowlinson, K. and Kempson, E. (1994) *Paying with Plastic: A Study of Credit Card Debt.* London: Policy Studies Institute.

Russell, J. and Gablik, S. (1969) *Pop Art Redefined.* London: Thames and Hudson.

Sabel, C.F. (1984) *Work and Politics: The Division of Labour in Industry.* Cambridge: Cambridge University Press (first published 1982).

Sartre, J-P. (1943) *Being and Nothingness: A Phenomenological Essay on Ontology.* New York: Philosophical Library.

Saunders, P. (1984) 'Beyond Housing Classes: The sociological significance of private property', *International Journal of Urban and Regional Research*, 8: 202–27.

Saunders, P. (1986) *Social Theory and the Urban Question*, (second edition). London: Hutchinson.

Saunders, P. (1988) 'The sociology of consumption: a new research agenda', in P. Otnes (ed.).

Saunders, P. (1990) *Social Class and Stratification.* London: Tavistock.

Saussure, F. de. (1966) *Course in General Linguistics.* New York.

Savage, M. (2000), *Class Analysis and Social Transformation.* Buckingham: Open University Press.

Savage, M., Barlow, J., Dickens, P. and Fielding, T. (1992) *Property, Bureaucracy and Culture: Middle-class Formation in Contemporary Britain.* London: Routledge.

Sayers, S. (1987) 'The need to work', *Radical Philosophy*, 46: 17–26. Reprinted in R.E. Pahl (ed.), 1988. pp. 722–41.

Sayers, S. (1998) *Marxism and Human Nature*, (Routledge Studies in Social and Political Thought). New York: Routledge.

Schor, J. (1991) *The Overworked American: The Unexpected Decline of Leisure.* New York: Basic Books.

Schor, J. (1998) *The Overspent American.* New York: Harper Perennial.

Schumpeter, J.A. (1989) *Essays on Entrepreneurs, Innovations, Business Cycles, and the Evolution of Capitalism*, R.V. Clemenc (ed.). Oxford: Transaction Publishers.

Schwimmer, E. (1979) 'The self and the product: concepts of work in comparative perspective', in S. Wallman (ed.). pp. 287–315.

Scott, A.M. (ed.) (1994) *Gender Segregation and Social Change: Men and Women in Changing Labour Markets.* Oxford: Oxford University Press.

Scott, J. (1996) *Stratification and Power: Structures of Class, Status and Command.* Cambridge: Polity Press.

Sen, A. (1998) 'The living standard', in Crocker, D.A. and Linden, T. (eds). pp. 287–311. Reproduced in D. Millar (ed.) 2001c, Vol. I. pp. 406–28.

Seidler, V.J. (1989) *Rediscovering Masculinity: Reason, Language and Sexuality.* London: Routledge.

Seidler, V.J. (ed.) (1991) *The Achilles Heel Reader: Men, Sexual Politics and Socialism.* London: Routledge.